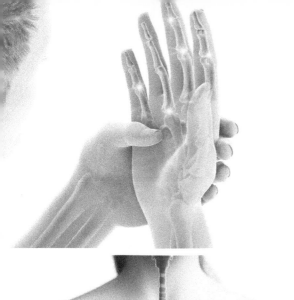

Long-term Conditions in Adults

at a Glance

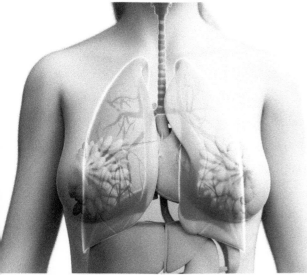
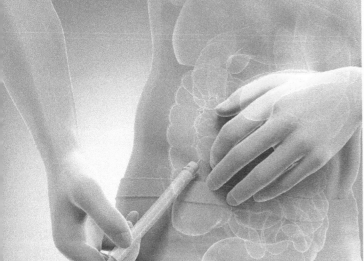
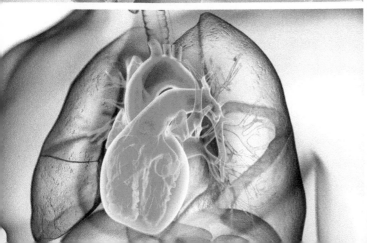

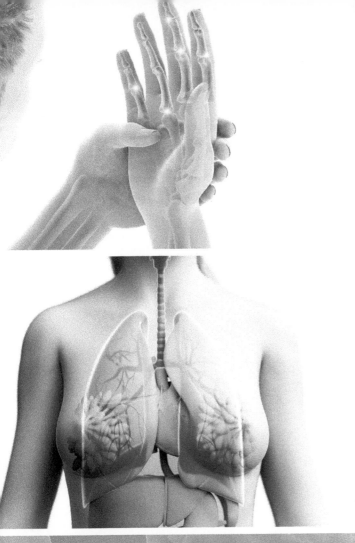
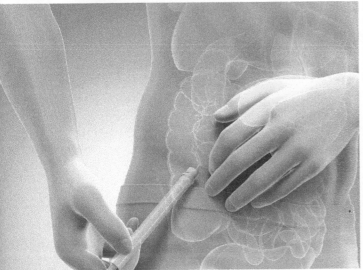
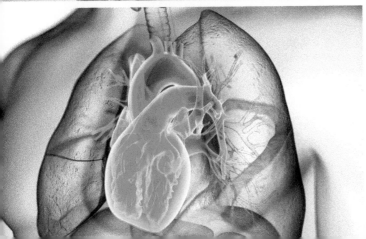

Long-term Conditions in Adults

at a Glance

Edited by

Aby Mitchell RGN, MSc, PGCert, BA, FHEA
Senior Lecturer in Nursing Education,
Department of Adult Nursing, Florence
Nightingale Faculty of Nursing, Midwifery,
and Palliative Care, King's College London

**Barry Hill MSc Adv Prac, PGCAP,
BSc (Hons) CCRN, DipHE/O.A. Dip, SFHEA,
TEFL, NMC RN RNT/TCH V300**
Associate Professor, Nursing Science and
Critical Care; Director of Employability,
Northumbria University, UK

Ian Peate OBE FRCN
Editor in Chief British Journal of Nursing.
Visiting Professor St Georges University of
London and Kingston University London;
Visiting Professor Northumbria University;
Professorial Fellow Roehampton University;
Visiting Senior Clinical Fellow University of
Hertfordshire

WILEY Blackwell

This edition first published 2023
© 2023 by John Wiley & Sons Ltd

The right of Aby Mitchell, Barry Hill, and Ian Peate to be identified as the authors of the editorial material in this work has been asserted in accordance with law.

Registered Offices
John Wiley & Sons, Inc., 111 River Street, Hoboken, NJ 07030, USA
John Wiley & Sons Ltd, The Atrium, Southern Gate, Chichester, West Sussex, PO19 8SQ, UK

For details of our global editorial offices, customer services, and more information about Wiley products visit us at www.wiley.com.

Wiley also publishes its books in a variety of electronic formats and by print-on-demand. Some content that appears in standard print versions of this book may not be available in other formats.

Library of Congress Cataloging-in-Publication Data
Names: Mitchell, Aby, editor. | Hill, Barry (Lecturer in nursing), editor.
  | Peate, Ian, editor.
Title: Long-term conditions in adults at a glance / Aby Mitchell, Barry
  Hill, Ian Peate.
Other titles: At a glance series (Oxford, England)
Description: First edition. | Hoboken, NJ : Wiley-Blackwell, 2023. |
  Series: At a glance series | Includes bibliographical references and
  index.
Identifiers: LCCN 2023000297 (print) | LCCN 2023000298 (ebook) | ISBN
  9781119875871 (paperback) | ISBN 9781119875888 (adobe pdf) | ISBN
  9781119875895 (epub)
Subjects: MESH: Chronic Disease | Adult | Socioeconomic Factors | Life
  Style | Patient Education as Topic | Self-Management | Handbook
Classification: LCC RB127 (print) | LCC RB127 (ebook) | NLM QZ 39 | DDC
  616/.0478–dc23/eng/20230516
LC record available at https://lccn.loc.gov/2023000297
LC ebook record available at https://lccn.loc.gov/2023000298

Cover Design: Wiley
Cover Image: © SEBASTIAN KAULITZKI/SCIENCE PHOTO LIBRARY/Getty Images;
SCIEPRO/Getty Images; SCIEPRO/SCIENCE PHOTO LIBRARY/Getty Images

Set in 9.5/11.5 pt MinionPro by Straive, Pondicherry, India
Printed and bound by CPI Group (UK) Ltd, Croydon, CR0 4YY
C9781119875871_291123

Contents

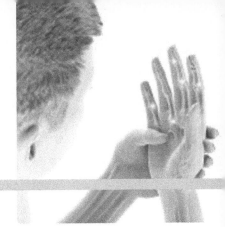

Contributors   viii
Preface   x

Part 1

Long-term conditions: sociological factors   1

1   Determinants of health   2
Daniela Blumlein and Ian Griffiths

2   Health inequalities   4
Ian Peate

3   Environmental factors   6
Giuseppe Leontino

4   Housing   10
Ian Peate

5   Public health   12
Ian Peate

6   Lifestyle factors   14
Ian Peate

7   Socioeconomic status   16
Ian Peate

8   Holistic needs assessment   18
Ian Peate

Part 2

Patient education and self-management   21

9   Behavioural change   22
Barry Hill

10   Health education: developing a partnership with patients with long-term conditions   24
Pamela Arasen

11   Patient responsibility   26
Ian Peate

12   Self-care and self-management   28
Barry Hill

13   Effectively supporting carers   30
Rachael Betty

14   Empowerment in long-term conditions   32
Sara Tavares

15   Experts by experience   34
Sue Tiplady

Part 3 Long-term conditions 37

16 Alcohol dependency 38
Leticia Wedderburn and Helen Phillips

17 Anorexia nervosa 40
Tichaona Mubaira

18 Arthritis 42
Emily Ashwell

19 Asthma 44
Barry Hill

20 Angina 46
Barry Hill

21 Anxiety 48
Louise Lingwood

22 Atrial fibrillation 50
Barry Hill

23 Bipolar affective disorder 52
Vishal Jugessur and Angela Childs

24 Bulimia nervosa 54
Tichaona Mubaira and Lucy Saunders

25 Bronchiectasis 56
Barry Hill

26 Cancer 58
Ian Peate

27 Chronic fatigue syndrome 60
Roberta Borg

28 Chronic venous insufficiency 62
Aby Mitchell

29 Chronic obstructive pulmonary disease (COPD) 66
Barry Hill

30 Coronary artery Disease 68
Sadie Diamond-Fox

31 Chronic liver disease 70
Sadie Diamond-Fox

32 Depression 72
Sarah Bisp and Louise Lingwood

33 Diabetes mellitus type 1 74
Charlotte Gordon

34 Diabetes mellitus type 2 78
Charlotte Gordon

35 Dual diagnosis 82
Leticia Wedderburn and Daren Bailey

36 Diverticular disease 84
Laura Park and Claire Ford

37 Epilepsy 88
Ian Peate

38 Heart failure   90
Barry Hill

39 HIV   92
Ian Peate

40 Hypertension   94
Barry Hill

41 Inflammatory bowel disease   96
Claire Ford and Laura Park

42 Multiple sclerosis   98
Barry Hill

43 Parkinson's disease   100
Kelley Storey and Annette Hand

44 Peripheral arterial disease   102
Aby Mitchell

45 Psoriasis   104
Ian Peate

46 Rheumatoid arthritis   106
Jane Douglas and Karl Nicholl

47 Sickle cell   108
Barry Hill

48 Schizophrenia   110
Reuben Pearce and Helen Robson

49 Vascular dementia   112
Ian Peate

50 Viral hepatitis   114
Ian Peate

51 Visual impairment   116
Caitlin Gallon and Claire Ford

Part 4 Management of long-term conditions   119

52 Frameworks of care delivery – new ways of working   120
Barry Hill

53 Evidence-based practice   122
Claire Anderson

54 Leadership and management   124
Barry Hill

55 Chronic pain management   126
Claire Ford and Laura Park

56 End of life care   130
Jemma-Louise McCann and Sara Sinclair

57 Advanced care planning   132
Sara Sinclair

Bibliography   134
Index   140

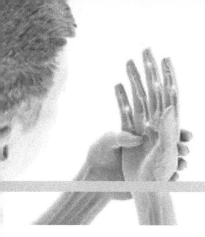

Contributors

Claire Anderson [Chapter 53]
Interim Deputy Dean Berkshire, College of Nursing Midwifery and Healthcare,
University of West London, London

Pamela Arasen [Chapter 10]
Senior Lecturer in Critical Care Nursing,
University of West London (UWL), London

Emily Ashwell [Chapter 18]
Community Case Manager Nurse,
Buckinghamshire Healthcare NHS Trust

Daren Bailey [Chapter 35]
Crisis Resolution and Home Treatment Team Hub Manager, Berkshire Healthcare NHS Foundation Trust

Rachael Betty [Chapter 13]
RMHN and Trainee Academic Advisor for the Accredited Learning Centre; Cumbria, Northumberland, Tyne and Wear NHS Foundation Trust

Sarah Bisp [Chapter 32]
Lecturer Mental Health Nursing,
Northumbria University, Newcastle

Daniela Blumlein [Chapter 1]
Senior Lecturer in Adult Nursing,
University of West London, London

Roberta Borg [Chapter 27]
Advanced Critical Care Practitioner (ACCP),
The Newcastle upon Tyne Hospitals NHS
Foundation Trust

Angela Childs [Chapter 23]
Specialist Clinical Mental Health Practitioner/Deputy Service Manager East Berkshire CRHT

Sadie Diamond-Fox [Chapter 30]
Strategic Lead for Advanced Practice Programmes and Assistant Professor in Advanced Critical Care Practice at Northumbria University,

Advanced Critical Care Practitioner at Newcastle upon Tyne Hospitals and Supervision and Assessment Lead for Advanced Critical Care Practice at Health Education England North East and Yorkshire

Jane Douglas [Chapter 46]
Assistant Professor, Adult Nursing,
Northumbria University, Newcastle

Claire Ford [Chapter 51]
Programme Lead for MSc Nursing and
Assistant Professor Adult Nursing, Northumbria University, Newcastle

Caitlin Gallon [Chapter 51]
Registered Nurse in Ophthalmology, The Newcastle upon Tyne Hospitals NHS Foundation Trust

Charlotte Gordon [Chapter 34]
Assistant Professor, Adult Nursing,
Northumbria University, Newcastle

Ian Griffiths [Chapter 1]
Senior Staff Nurse, Medical Infusions,
Royal Berkshire NHS Foundation Trust

Annette Hand [Chapter 43]
Clinical Academic Professor of Nursing
at Northumbria University, Newcastle

Barry Hill [Chapters 9, 12, 19, 20, 22, 25, 29, 38, 40, 42, 47, 52, 54]
Associate Professor, Nursing Science and
Critical Care; Director of Employability,
Northumbria University, UK

Vishal Jugessur [Chapter 23]
Service Manager Crisis Resolution Home
Treatment Team, Registered Mental Health Nurse and Nonmedical Prescriber, Berkshire Healthcare
Foundation Trust

Giuseppe Leontino [Chapter 3]
Senior Lecturer in Simulation and
Immersive Technologies, University of West London, London

Louise Lingwood [Chapter 3]
Assistant Professor in Mental Health Nursing at
Northumbria University, Newcastle

Jemma-Louise McCann [Chapter 56]
Advanced Clinical Practitioner / District Nurse,
Non-medical Prescriber, Community Practice
Teacher, Berkshire Healthcare Foundation Trust

Aby Mitchell [Chapter 28]
Senior Lecturer in Nursing Education, Department of
Adult Nursing, Florence Nightingale Faculty of Nursing,
Midwifery, and Palliative Care, King's College London

Tichaona Mubaira [Chapters 17, 24]
Clinical Nurse Specialist, Crisis Resolution and
Home Treatment Services, Berkshire Healthcare NHS
Foundation Trust and
Associate Lecturer, University of West London, London

Karl Nicholl [Chapter 46]
Biologics Nurse Specialist in Rheumatology,
the Freeman Hospital, Newcastle upon Tyne

Laura Park [Chapters 36, 55]
Lecturer, Adult Nursing,
Northumbria University, Newcastle

Reuben Pearce [Chapter 48]
Nurse Consultant, Crisis and Home Treatment Services,
Berkshire Healthcare NHS Foundation Trust and
Associate Lecturer, University of West London, London

Ian Peate [Chapters 2, 4–8, 11, 26, 37, 39, 45, 49, 50]
Editor in Chief British Journal of Nursing. Visiting Professor
St Georges University of London and Kingston University
London; Visiting Professor Northumbria University;
Professorial Fellow Roehampton University; Visiting
Senior Clinical Fellow University of Hertfordshire

Helen Phillips [Chapter 16]
Drug Alcohol and Smokefree Lead,
Mental Health Inpatients, Berkshire Healthcare

Helen Robson [Chapter 48]
Nurse Consultant, Inpatient MH Services,
Berkshire Healthcare Foundation Trust

Lucy Saunders [Chapter 24]
Assistant Psychologist and
QMIS/Carers Co-ordinator at Crisis Resolution and
Home Treatment Team (CRHTT) West, Berkshire
Healthcare NHS Foundation Trust

Sara Sinclair [Chapters 56, 57]
SPQ District Nursing Team Leader,
Berkshire Health Foundation Trust

Kelley Storey [Chapter 43]
Parkinson's Disease Nurse Specialist,
Newcastle upon Tyne Hospitals NHS Foundation Trust

Sara Tavares [Chapter 14]
Heart Failure Specialist Nurse, Non-medical Prescriber
and Immersive Technologies at University of West London,
London

Sue Tiplady [Chapter 15]
Assistant Professor Nursing Science,
Northumbria University, Newcastle upon Tyne

Leticia Wedderburn [Chapters 16, 35]
Urgent Care Dual Diagnosis Coordinator and
Psychological Medicine Practice Development Nurse,
Wexham Park Hospital, Berkshire

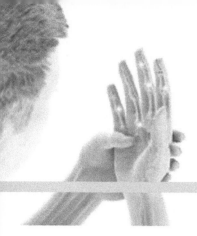

Preface

In the 70 years since the founding of the NHS, life expectancy has increased by around 13 years. But different types of diseases are becoming more common. More people are living with cancer or dementia largely due to increases in life expectancy and falls in the rate of premature death. With advances in prevention and medical care the UK mortality rate from heart and circulatory diseases has declined by more than three quarters in the last 40 years. But cardiovascular disease remains the biggest cause of premature mortality and the rate of improvement has slowed. Long-term conditions or chronic diseases are conditions for which there is currently no cure, and which are managed with drugs and other treatment, for example: diabetes mellitus, chronic obstructive pulmonary disease, arthritis, and hypertension. Longer-term health conditions also make an increasing contribution to the overall burden of disease. Mental health, respiratory and musculoskeletal conditions are responsible for a substantial amount of poor health and place a substantial burden on the NHS and other care services. The latest Global Burden of Disease study shows that the top five causes of early death for the people of England are: heart disease and stroke, cancer, respiratory conditions, dementias, and self-harm. It also reveals that the slower improvement since 2010 in years-of-life-lost is mainly driven by distinct condition-specific trends, predominantly in cardiovascular diseases and some cancers.

There are currently 15.4 million people in England with an LTC. Due to an ageing population, it is estimated that by 2025 there will be 42% more people in England aged 65 or over. This will mean that the number of people with at least one LTC will rise by 3–18 million. People with LTCs account for a significant and growing proportion of health and social care resources. The Department of Health's best estimate is that the treatment and care of people with LTCs account for 70% of the total health and social care spend in England, or almost £7 in every £10 spent. Social care expenditure, too, is focused on those with LTCs and will be put under pressure by the ageing population. By 2022 the proportion of those aged 65 and over will increase by 37% to 10.8 million; the number of people aged 65 and over with some disability will increase by 40% to 3.3 million; the number of disabled older people receiving informal care (in households) will rise by 39% to 2.4 million; the number of people in residential care homes will increase by 40% to 280 000; and the number of people in nursing homes will increase by 42% to 170 000. This need for social care will mean that by 2022 public expenditure on long-term care will rise by 94% to £15.9 billion. The total long-term care expenditure is forecast to rise by 29% to £26.4 billion. This is equivalent to a rise from 1.4% to 1.8% of GDP.

Health-care professionals are in a key position to support patients with long-term conditions attain a better quality of life through purposeful interventions that aim to minimise symptoms, reduce the intensity and frequency of acute exacerbations of the disease and enhance psycho-social well-being. Several public consultations such as 'Independence, Well-being and Choice' (GOV.UK) and 'Your Health, Your Care, Your Say' (NHS) have provided consistent messages from people with long-term conditions about what is important to them. Overall, people say they want services that support them to remain as independent and healthy as possible. They want increased choice, with information to help them make choices and to understand and manage their conditions better. They want far more services delivered safely and effectively in the community or at home, with more seamless, proactive, and integrated services that are personalised to them and their needs.

Long-term conditions: sociological factors

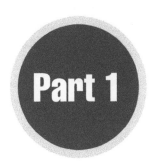

Part 1

Chapters

1 Determinants of health   2
2 Health inequalities   4
3 Environmental factors   6
4 Housing   10
5 Public health   12
6 Lifestyle factors   14
7 Socioeconomic status   16
8 Holistic needs assessment   18

Determinants of health

Daniela Blumlein and Ian Griffiths

Figure 1.1   The Rainbow model. Source: Dahlgren and Whitehead 1991.

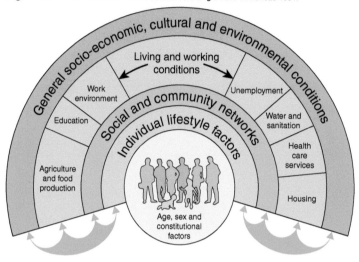

Table 1.1   Examples of Health Determinants

Category	Examples of Health Determinants
Biological Factors	Age, sex, inherited illnesses, genetics, co-morbidities, old age
Personal Lifestyle Factors	Smoking, obesity, alcohol consumption, substance abuse, level of physical activity
Social and Community Networks	Family connections, circle of friends, social isolation, loneliness
Living and Working Conditions	Employment status, level of education, access to clean water, sanitation, healthcare services, quality of housing, exposure to pollution, food production methods
Socioeconomic, Cultural, and Environmental Conditions	Conflicts and wars, droughts, floods, climate crisis, crime, economic issues like recessions and inflation, food security, pandemics

Long-term Conditions in Adults at a Glance, First Edition. Edited by Aby Mitchell, Barry Hill, and Ian Peate.
© 2023 John Wiley & Sons Ltd. Published 2023 by John Wiley & Sons Ltd.

Determinants of Health

This chapter explores the intricate concept of health determinants, endeavouring to establish an understanding of how various influences can impact and shape an individual's health trajectory throughout their lifespan. The concept of health extends far beyond the absence of illness; it is a state of complete physical, mental, and social well-being. Health is a resource for everyday life, not merely the objective of living, which underscores the importance of health determinants.

When we discuss an individual's well-being and health, it necessitates more than the absence of a specific illness or health disorder, whether physical or mental. The holistic health and well-being of a person are influenced by an assortment of known factors. These elements can generate either positive or negative effects on a person's physical or mental health and are generally recognised as 'determinants of health'.

Among the seminal models in understanding these determinants is the Rainbow model (Figure 1.1). Despite its years of inception, this model remains to be a cornerstone in health discussions and is widely applied today. It offers a comprehensive framework outlining how external and internal factors, along with various root causes, can significantly impact a person's overall health and well-being.

The Impact of Determinants of Health

Health inequalities persist as a global challenge, making their presence felt in almost every country around the world. The living conditions of an individual, influenced by an array of societal factors, significantly contribute to these disparities, directly and indirectly affecting their health outcomes.

Researchers and health professionals have identified various determinants of health (Table 1.1), with the following being some of the most pivotal:

1 **Biological factors:** Age, sex, and constitutional factors such as inherited illnesses and genetics play a crucial role. Co-morbidities or the inevitability of old age can significantly influence health outcomes.

2 **Personal lifestyle factors:** Health is greatly influenced by personal behaviours and habits. Factors such as smoking, obesity, alcohol consumption, substance abuse, or the level of physical activity can determine a person's health trajectory.

3 **Social and community networks:** The importance of social and community connections is paramount. A strong support system in the form of family, friends or a social circle can contribute positively to health outcomes, whereas loneliness and social isolation can have the opposite effect.

4 **Living and working conditions:** A person's living and working conditions are significant health determinants. They include elements such as employment status, level of education, access to clean water, sanitation and healthcare services, housing quality, exposure to pollution, and food production methods.

5 **Socioeconomic, cultural, and environmental conditions:** Wider societal issues, including conflicts and wars, droughts, floods, climate crisis, crime, economic turbulence such as recessions and inflation, food security, and pandemics, also bear heavily on health.

The Rainbow model shifts the focus onto these wider aspects that may influence an individual's health. It moves beyond a strictly medicalised model, which often centres on treating an illness without addressing its wider causes or potential preventative measures. This broader perspective is crucial as it allows policy makers and healthcare professionals to collaborate closely with other professionals, developing strategies that provide a structured pathway to addressing each of the determinants of health.

For instance, if substandard housing conditions emerge as a significant issue, a broad range of professionals may be called upon to address the problem. This multidisciplinary team might involve architects, housing officers, healthcare professionals, police forces, environmental services, and community representatives.

Another way to consider health determinants is through a comparison of individuals living in starkly contrasting environments. Consider a person residing in a war-torn country, confronted with the daily realities of violence, fear, and famine, against someone living in a peaceful country, with ready access to a variety of foods and high-quality healthcare services. The overall well-being of these two individuals would be remarkably different, largely influenced by the determinants of health.

The task of addressing these health inequalities and ensuring equal access to healthcare services is paramount and complex. Policy makers shoulder a substantial responsibility to legislate for a more equitable society. In the UK, attempts have been made towards this through the implementation of the Care Act (Department of Health, 2014) and the NHS 10-Year Long Term Plan (NHS, 2018). These measures aim to enhance access to services and support individuals in maintaining good health throughout their lifespan. Ensuring these services are provided at every life stage, from prenatal to end-of-life care, is crucial.

A comprehensive understanding of the determinants of health is instrumental in forging policies and strategies aimed at improving population health and reducing health inequalities. By exploring the breadth and depth of these determinants, we open avenues for intervention, prevention, and health promotion, ultimately empowering individuals, and communities to achieve optimal health and well-being.

Health inequalities

2

Ian Peate

Figure 2.1 Equity, access, human rights, and participation; the four essential principles underpinning social justice.

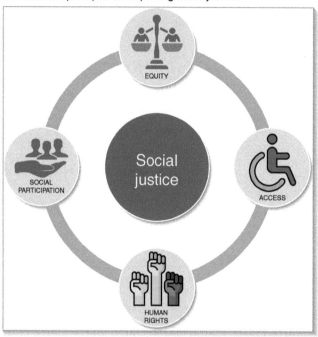

Table 2.1 Selected impacts of wider determinants on health and well-being. Source: Adapted from Williams et al. 2020.

Sector	Examples
Income	Income has the potential to determine a person's ability to buy health-improving goods, for example, food to membership to a gym. Attempting to cope on a low income is a cause of stress and it can also affect the way people make choices regarding health affecting behaviours
Housing	Overcrowded housing and poor-quality housing stock are correlated with an increased risk of cardiovascular diseases, respiratory diseases, depression as well as anxiety. In those colder homes, when external temperature falls, death rates increase much faster. Households from minority ethnic groups are more likely than white households to live in overcrowded homes and to experience fuel poverty.
Environment	Being able to access to good-quality green space has been associated with improvements in physical and mental health as well as decreased levels of obesity. Those in deprived areas and in those areas with higher proportions of minority ethnic groups have poorer levels of access to green spaces. Exposure to air pollutants has been linked to deprivation and ethnicity. Within the most deprived areas of London, for example, people from non-white groups have been found to be more exposed to higher concentrations of one of the main pollutants associated with traffic fumes – nitrogen oxide.
Transport	People who are living in the most deprived areas have a 50% greater risk of dying in road accident than those living the in the least deprived areas. Children in deprived areas are four times more likely to be killed or injured on the road than those in wealthier areas.
Education	People with a university degree or an equivalent level of education at age 30 years can expect to live more than 5 years longer than those with lower levels of education.
Work	Lower life expectancy, poorer physical, and also mental health are linked with unemployment for individuals who are unemployed and also for those in their households. The quality of work and this includes exposure to hazards, job security, and whether the job/type of work promotes a sense of belonging, impacts physical, and mental health.

The social determinants of health are the broad social and economic circumstances that when brought together can influence a person's health throughout their lives (see Chapter 1). A number of these determinants that contribute to health can result in health inequalities with those people who are poorer experiencing worse health outcomes than those who are better off.

Social justice

Social justice is concerned with making society function better. It is about fairness, fairness in health care, employment, housing and more, providing people with the support and the tools they need to help them turn their lives around with a focus on prevention and early intervention. Where problems emerge, there needs to be a focus on interventions related to recovery and independence as opposed to maintenance. Social justice and discrimination are incompatible concepts. There are a number of key drivers that underpin any social justice strategy, for example, wealth, education, privilege, opportunities, and health.

There are four essential principles associated with social justice (see Figure 2.1). Without these four principles social justice cannot be achieved: human rights, access, participation, and equity.

Reducing health inequalities is seen as a driving force for the NHS and Public Health as the best evidence of how health is improving; it is however complex. There are many causes of health inequalities; few of these causes are directly related to the provision of health and social care. Health inequalities are irrefutably related to social justice.

The lower a person's social position, the worse their health outcomes are likely to be. Health inequalities cannot be attributed simply to genes, unhealthy behaviour, or difficulties in access to medical care, important as those factors may be. There is often a tendency to apportion 'blame' to individuals and groups, but the reality is far more complex.

Health inequalities

Health inequalities are avoidable and unfair differences in health status that occur between groups of people or communities. They can include inequality in health outcomes by socioeconomic status or level of deprivation or by characteristics, for example, gender, ethnic group, or sexual orientation. Some individuals and families face multiple disadvantages and they do not always receive the support that they need, when they need it.

Health inequalities are avoidable, unfair, and systematic differences in health between different groups of people. There are many kinds of health inequality, and many ways in which the term is used. This means that when we talk about 'health inequality', it is useful to be clear on which measure is unequally distributed, and between which people.

When discussing health inequality it is essential that all aspects of health, including physical, mental and emotional are addressed. The concept of 'well-being' must also be given consideration. A person may have a incapacitating long-term condition, however, they may be enjoy a satisfying life; similarly a person could appear to be in good physical health but they may lack the desire and enthusiasm to achieve their full potential (whatever this is for them).

Impact of health inequalities

The term health inequalities is often used to also make reference to differences in the care that individuals receive and the opportunities they have in order to lead healthy lives. Both can influence a person's health status. Health inequalities can be associated with differences in:

• health status, for example, life expectancy and frequency of health conditions
• accessing care, for example, availability of treatments
• quality and experience of care, for example, levels of patient satisfaction
• behavioural risks to health, for example, smoking rates
• wider determinants of health, for example, quality of accommodation.

Variations in health status and those factors that determine it can be experienced by people who are grouped with respect to a variety of issues. Often, health inequalities can be analysed and addressed by cross cutting policy:

• such as socioeconomic factors, for example, income
• geography, for example, region or whether urban or rural
• particular characteristics including those that are protected in law, such as sex, ethnicity, or disability
• those groups who are socially excluded, for example, people who experience homelessness.

The wider determinants of health

The wider determinants of health are the social, economic, and environmental conditions in which people live that have an impact on their health. These include income, education, access to green space and healthy food, the work that people do and the homes in which live in.

When taken together, these factors are the key drivers of how healthy people are and that any inequalities in these factors will be a fundamental reason for health inequality. In reducing health inequalities therefore, it is paramount to address the wider social–economic inequalities. In Table 2.1 a number of examples are given regarding health impacts concerning the wider determinants. In the examples provided they emphasise the individual determinants; these determinants however are frequently experienced together and increase over time.

Relieving the effects of health inequalities

Actions that are more likely to be successful in relieving the effects of health inequalities at an individual level will require a revision of public services and health-care professionals must have a significant input in any change. Redesign of public services will include targeting high-risk individuals, and intensive personalised support for those who have most need, along with a focus on early child development.

Stark health inequalities remain and they continue to damage the lives of many people locally, nationally and internationally. There are some groups of people who die much earlier and spend more of their life in ill health than others. This is not happening by chance. These health inequalities are the result of a range of social, economic, and environment factors essentially beyond people's individual control. This is unjust and unfair. They are not inevitable and they can be reversed. All of us should have the opportunity to live a long life, in good health.

Environmental factors

3

Giuseppe Leontino

Figure 3.1 Long-term conditions in numbers. England.

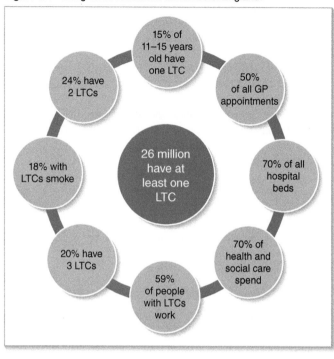

Table 3.1 Long-term conditions and main risk factors.
Source: Available from https://www.sciencedirect.com/science/article/pii/S2214999616000059#appsec1

Disease	Exposure
Asthma	• Tobacco smoke • Ambient/household air pollution • Ecological exposure to PCBs
COPD	• Tobacco smoke • Ambient/household air pollution • Ecological exposure to PCBs • POPs • Gastrointestinal dysbiosis
Cancer	• Ambient air pollution • Arsenic • POPs
CVDs	• Tobacco smoke • POPs • Ambient air pollution • Household air pollution • Ambient noise
T2D	• POPs • Bisphenol A/phthalates • Ambient air pollution
HYP	• Tobacco smoke • POPs • Ambient air pollution • Arsenic (drinking water)
Neurodegenerative disorder	• Heavy metals • Air pollution • Herbicides

Figure 3.2 Prevalence of long-term conditions in England. AF, atrial fibrillation; HF, heart failure; HYP, hypertension; STIA, stroke and ischaemic attack; CHD, coronary heart disease; COPD, chronic obstructive pulmonary disease; AST, asthma; CAN, cancer; CKD, chronic kidney disease; DM, diabetes mellitus; DEM, dementia; DEP, depression; EP, epilepsy; LD, learning disability; MH, mental health; OST, osteoporosis; RA, rheumatoid arthritis.

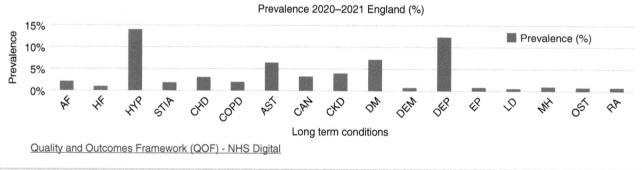

Long-term conditions (LTCs) are chronic health conditions that do not have a cure but that can be managed by medications or other therapies. Figure 3.1 gives a snapshot of the current situation in England whilst Figure 3.2 provides an insight around prevalence of LTCs.

The World Health Organization (WHO) produced evidence that ascribed 24% of the global disease and 23% of all deaths to long-term environmental exposures in adults, and up to 36% in children aged 0–14 years old.

The environment is made of different elements that contribute to improving and diminishing people's health depending on accessibility to:
• clean air and water
• transportation

- green spaces and cycle lanes
- wellness facilities.

Environmental health is concerned with elements of the environment that are directly affected by human activities like man-made structures, and those linked to the intrinsic meaning of nature itself like geography. Geographical characteristics influence the climate and the resources available to people. For instance, direct sunlight exposure promotes healthy levels of vitamin D. In the United Kingdom (UK) 34% of men and 33% of women have been found to be deficient in this rather life-essential hormone. In fact, the UK has lower overall vitamin D status compared to Western Europe. Levels of vitamin D < 25 nmol/l can lead to:

- rickets
- osteomalacia
- osteoporosis.

The recommended levels of vitamin D of more than 50 nmol/l can be maintained by fortifying foods like wheat flour or supplementation:

- 8.5–10 μg of vitamin D a day for babies up to the age of one years old
- 10 μg of vitamin D a day for children from the age of one years old and adults.

Physical factors

LTCs may originate from an inflammatory response mechanism derived from consistent and prolonged exposure to toxins present in all aspects of the physical environment:

- soil
- aquatic
- atmospheric
- built ecosystems.

These toxins originate from a plethora of sources such as:

- vehicles and fuels
- Industries and factories.

Some of the pollutants currently identified as highly injurious to health are:

- tobacco smoke
- traffic-related pollutants
- polycyclic aromatic hydrocarbons
- endocrine-disrupting chemicals
- heavy metals
- UV and ionising radiations
- dioxins, furans
- bioaerosols
- phytoestrogens
- tributyltin (TBT)
- bisphenol A (BPA)
- diethylstilbesterol (DES).

The effects of long-term exposure even at low dosage to these pollutants may lead to a variety of conditions as shown in Table 3.1.

Studies addressing the ever-growing rate of metabolic diseases suggest that these are not solely caused by:

- food choices
- genetic predisposition
- physical exercise.

There is strong evidence to suggest that air pollutants and endocrine disrupting chemicals could be linked to metabolic disorders such as diabetes and obesity. The mechanisms of action are multiple:

- lipid and glucose metabolism
- endothelium inflammation

- altering homeostatic metabolic set-points
- disrupting appetite controls
- direct binding to nuclear receptors acting as agonists or antagonists
- enzymatic activity inhibition.

Areas with high levels of small particulate matter (PM 2.5) have been linked to a worsening of symptoms in people who suffer from respiratory disorders, resulting in increased hospital admissions and about 5% of total mortality in England. PM 2.5 and nitrogen dioxide (NO_2) together account for a health annual cost of around £22.6 billion. The exposure to these toxins has been reduced by 44% and 56% respectively between 1970 and 2010.

After air pollutants, noises have been classified as the second largest environmental toxin in Western Europe. Noise pollution has been determined to be more detrimental to health than lead, ozone, and dioxins. The main source of noise pollution is road traffic which affects 11.5 million in England.

Noise pollution has been linked to:

- severe chronic annoyance
- coronary heart disease
- metabolic conditions, such as diabetes and obesity
- disruption to children's learning and development.

Sleep disturbance promotes long-term consequences in healthy individuals by affecting the:

- sympathetic nervous system
- hypothalamic–pituitary–adrenal axis
- metabolic syndrome
- changes in circadian rhythms
- proinflammatory responses.

These effects can in the long term lead to:

- hypertension
- dyslipidaemia
- cardiovascular disease
- weight-related issues
- metabolic syndrome
- type 2 diabetes mellitus
- colorectal cancer.

One study has estimated the medical cost of noise-related hypertension and associated conditions in the UK at £1.09 billion a year. The findings suggested that exposure to noise above recommended levels resulted in an extra:

- 1169 cases of dementia
- 788 strokes
- 542 heart attacks.

The total social cost of road traffic noise pollution, including health costs, productivity losses and chronic severe annoyance, has been estimated to be more than £9 billion annually.

Psycho-social factors

The social environment can be as harmful as air pollution. Psycho-social factors are responsible for inducing mental health disorders as well as physical health conditions.

The social environment includes factors such as:

- safety
- occupation
- criminal activity and violence
- social connections
- social participation
- social cohesion
- social capital.

Mental health disorders have been linked to increased levels of stress that derives from:

* safety
* social disorders
* social participation
* integration.

Conversely, the quality of social connections and social support may improve health by increasing resilience which buffers the adverse effect of stress.

Occupational and socioeconomic risk factors have been investigated for the potential to develop and promote:

* inadequate physical activity
* drug and alcohol use
* labour-intense occupation
* exposure to dusts, silica, and other air pollutants.

Studies have reported the connection between self-reported health status and social capital which is defined as 'the network of relationships amongst individuals who live and work in a society, enabling that society to function effectively.' Furthermore, social capital interventions can endorse mental health well-being and prevent common mental health disorders (CMD) such as:

* depression
* generalised anxiety disorder (GAD)
* panic disorder
* phobias
* social anxiety disorder
* obsessive-compulsive disorder (OCD)
* post-traumatic stress disorder (PTSD).

Conclusions

Environmental exposure and behavioural risk factors act synergistically to promote ill-health. Therefore, lifestyle choices alone cannot deter the risk of developing LTCs. Education, government policies, research, and life-time choices should all be adopted to improve health and reduce the compound effect that may lead to LTCs.

Further research in the field of epidemiology and epigenetics could provide a better understanding and a stronger link between environmental factors and LTCs.

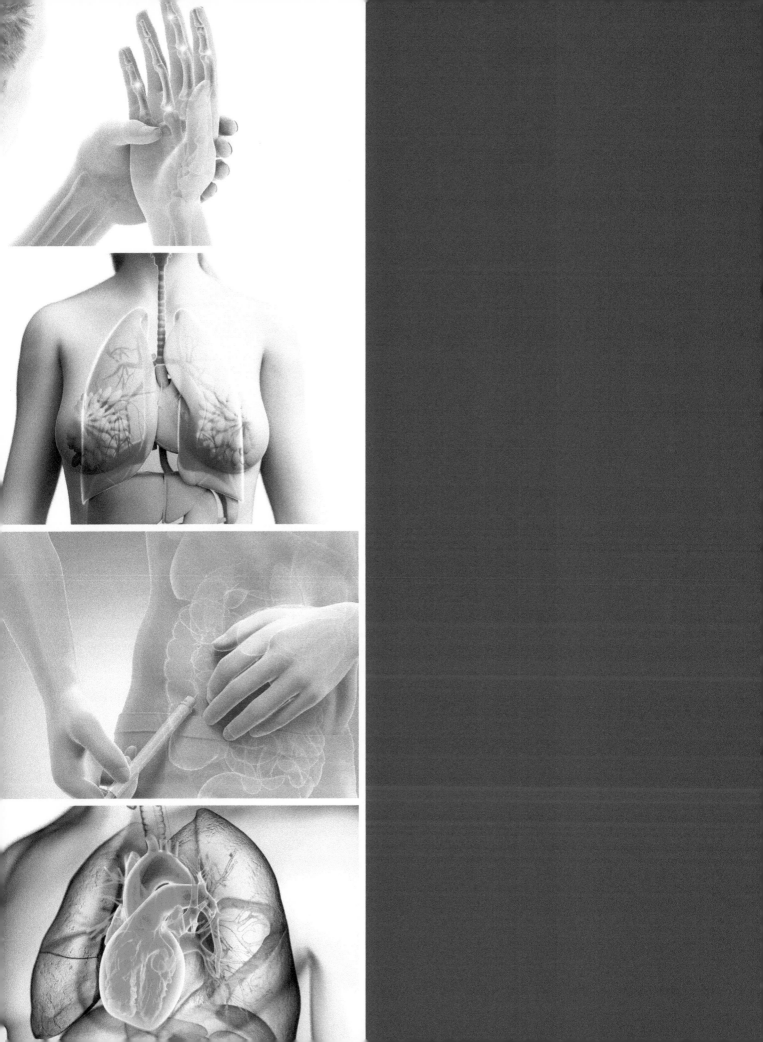

Housing

4

Ian Peate

Figure 4.1 Unhealthy, unsuitable and precarious housing. Source: PHE 2019.

Unhealthy homes increase the risk of

- respiratory illness
- cardiovascular problems
- excess winter deaths
- physical injuries, particularly from falls
- domestic fires

Unsuitable homes increase the risk of

- physical injuries, particularly from falls
- general health deterioration following a fall
- social isolation

Precarious housing and homelessness increases the risk of

- physical and mental health problems
- alcohol and drug misuse
- suicide
- tobacco harm
- tuberculosis

Underlying health issues can in turn raise the risk of being homeless or living in precarious housing

Table 4.1 An example of medical priority bands.

Priority band	Description
A: Emergency medical need	Band A is awarded to a person if it is deemed that the household contains one or more members with a currently life-threatening illness or disability and whose housing circumstances are impacting their health very severely.
B: Urgent medical need	In this band one member of the household or more has to have a serious illness or disability and their present living conditions are affecting their health to a significant degree and where a move is advised to improve the person's health.
C: Less urgent medical need	An individual is awarded band C if one or more in the household has an illness or disability that is moderate in nature which is negatively affected by the person's living conditions and where a move is recommended to enhance the health of the individual.
D: No medical need	This band will be awarded if a person has an illness or a disability where rehousing may improve the person's quality of life, the living conditions however are not thought to be significantly harmful to the person's health or functional ability.

Long-term Conditions in Adults at a Glance, First Edition. Edited by Aby Mitchell, Barry Hill, and Ian Peate.
© 2023 John Wiley & Sons Ltd. Published 2023 by John Wiley & Sons Ltd.

Poor housing conditions are associated with a wide range of health conditions, these include respiratory infections, asthma, injuries, and poor mental health. Addressing housing issues for those people with long-term conditions, provides health-care practitioners with an opportunity to address an important social determinant of health (see also Chapters 1 and 2). Substandard housing is a major public health issue.

The home

Housing is important for a number of aspects of healthy living and well-being. The home is important for psycho-social reasons as well as for the physical protection it offers against the extremes of weather. The home is the environment in which most people will spend the majority of their time. A home should not just be seen only as a roof over our head, it is also a safe, supportive place to live. Having a home which is safe and also affordable is very important for a person's health and well-being. If a person has poor housing or if they are homeless, this can increase the possibilities of them developing a mental health problem, or could make an existing mental health condition harder to manage.

The wider local environment that surrounds the home is also important with regards to fear of crime, the accessibility of services and the opportunity to be physically active. In unstable economic conditions, the affordability of housing and the potential for individuals to lose their home as a result of debts they are unable to meet is a problem for a large number of people.

Health and the home

A number of risks are present to an individual's physical and mental health associated with living in unhealthy home such as a cold, damp, or otherwise hazardous home, homes that do not meet the household's needs due to risks, such as, being overcrowded or inaccessible to a disabled or older people are unsuitable homes, these home bring with them inherent risks, an unstable home is one that does not provide the household with a sense of safety and security including dangerous living circumstances and/or homelessness. See Figure 4.1.

The right home environment as well as providing protection can enable people with long-term conditions to manage their own health and care needs, to live independently, safely and well in their own home for as long as they choose, to complete their treatment regimens and to recover from substance misuse, tuberculosis or other ill-health, to move on successfully from homelessness or other traumatic life events, to access and sustain education, training and employment and for participate and contribute to society.

The right home environment can also:
• delay and reduce the need for primary care and social care
• avoid hospital admissions
• facilitate timely discharge from hospital, and avoid re-admissions
• enable rapid recovery from periods of ill health or planned admissions.

Medical assessment: housing

Most councils/local authorities will give priority for social housing based on medical need aligned to their own regulations. Housing associations offer similar types of housing as local councils. Housing is often offered to those people who are on a low income or who need extra support. They also make recommendations about the type of property a person may need due to any disabilities or mobility requirements.

Table 4.1 provides an example of medical priority banding. In this example there are four medical priority bands, with band A being the highest and band D the lowest. A person can be placed in band A, B, C, or D for a number of medical and non-medical reasons. The overall priority band will be the highest band that they qualify for. If, for example, a person qualifies for band B due to overcrowding and band C as a result of medical need, the overall priority will be band B as this is the higher of the two.

Usually a person can apply for a priority move on medical grounds by applying for health and medical rehousing. Applicants must have a physical disability as defined in the Equality Act 2010 or a long-term medical condition that prevents them from accessing essential facilities within their home. This includes anyone who experiences excessive pain, substantial discomfort or difficulty in performing day to day tasks (these are common experiences in those with long-term conditions) and it can be proved that a move to a different property type will significantly relieve these difficulties. The Equality Act 2010 defines disability as physical (including sensory) or mental impairment which has had a 'substantial' or 'long-term' adverse effect upon a person's ability to perform normal day to day activities. Examples may include: difficulty getting in and out of their home; difficulty going up and downstairs; difficulty reaching the toilet; difficulty maintaining personal hygiene; and problems with lighting or heating that will affect their health.

When the assessment form has been completed a Medical Assessment Officer will make an assessment based on the application. There is no requirement for the applicant to seek a GP or hospital letter of support. If further information is required the assessment officer will contact the relevant people directly, i.e. GP.

Adapted housing

This refers to housing which is built for or adapted to suit, the needs of those people with long-term conditions in order to enable them to maintain an independent lifestyle. Good adaptations of a home can have a huge impact on well-being and quality of life, helping people stay in their home for longer. A home that is more suitable to meet a person's needs can help to make everyday tasks easier. Such housing may include:
• ceiling hoist
• level access
• level or stepped access shower
• full wheelchair access (including widened doorway)
• raised sockets
• stairlift
• kitchen adapted for a person using a wheelchair
• specialised fitted aids, such as, grab rails, hoists.

People with a long-term condition who need or feel they need adaptation to their existing property to enable them to continue to stay in their home are encouraged to seek advice from health-care professionals such as an occupational therapist, general practice nurse, GP, social worker, and landlord or housing services.

Public health

5

Ian Peate

Figure 5.1 Public Health Liverpool: targeted health campaign.

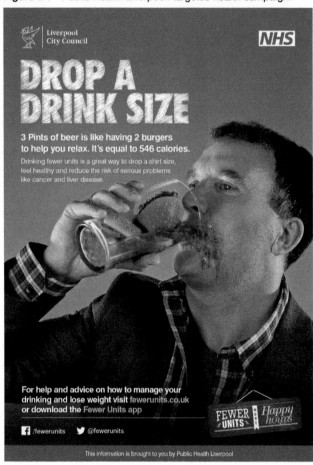

Figure 5.2 The 3 Ps and surveillance.

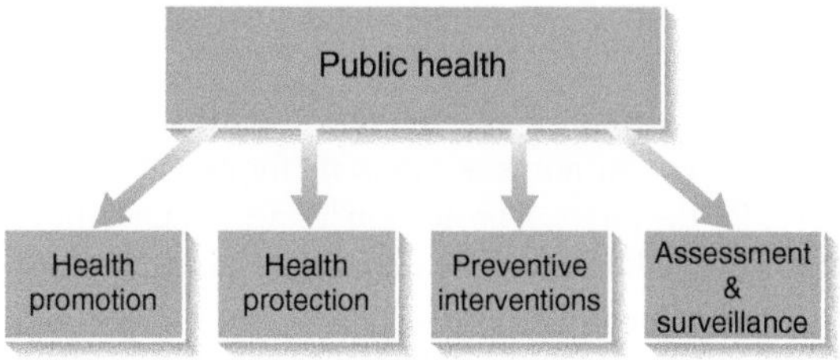

Public health

- Health promotion
- Health protection
- Preventive interventions
- Assessment & surveillance

Figure 5.3 Eight steps diagram for planning and implementing MECC. Source: Public Health England and Health Education England (2018a,b).

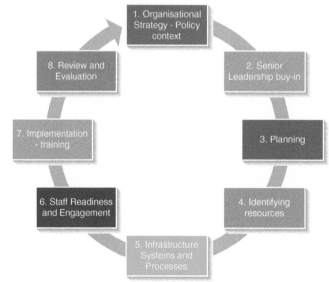

1. Organisational Strategy - Policy context
2. Senior Leadership buy-in
3. Planning
4. Identifying resources
5. Infrastructure Systems and Processes
6. Staff Readiness and Engagement
7. Implementation - training
8. Review and Evaluation

Long-term Conditions in Adults at a Glance, First Edition. Edited by Aby Mitchell, Barry Hill, and Ian Peate.
© 2023 John Wiley & Sons Ltd. Published 2023 by John Wiley & Sons Ltd.

Public health

In 1988 public health was defined as 'the art and science of preventing disease, prolonging life, and promoting health through the organised efforts of society' this definition still holds true today. Those activities that are undertaken to strengthen public health capacities and service aim to provide conditions under which people can maintain their health, improve their health and well-being or prevent deterioration of their health. Public health has a focus on the entire range of health and well-being, it is not only about the eradication of particular diseases. Many activities are targeted at populations such as health campaigns (see Figure 5.1). Public health services also include the provision of personal services to individuals, such as vaccinations, behavioural counselling or health advice, it refers to all organised measures (public or private) that set out to prevent disease, promote health and prolong life among the population as a whole.

Public health has a wide variety of valuable roles to play across sectors. These roles include developing and delivering vaccination programmes (including COVID-19 vaccinations), ensuring people have access to safe drinking water and food supplies, managing disease outbreaks, monitoring, and reporting on health status and encouraging healthy behaviours to prevent disease, disability, and injury. Public health activity impacts the age continuum from conception to death.

As the services provided by public health organisations is wide and varied so too are the public health officials who are providing these services. These include nurses, doctors, public health inspectors, nutritionists and dieticians, dental hygienists, vision screening technologists, mental health, and addictions specialists and a myriad of other healthcare professionals. With so many factors impacting public health (including the emergence and re-emergence of infectious diseases), an increasing awareness about health inequalities, long-term conditions, conditions associated with our ageing population and health related consequences of environmental factors, such as air pollution, a strong public health presence is as important today than it ever was.

Prevent, protect, and promote

Prevention of avoidable illness, health protection, and promotion of well-being and resilience are important areas where health and care professionals, regardless of their role, wherever it is they work can take action on the major health challenges that contemporary societies face. The 3 Ps of public health are seen as:

* preventing avoidable disease
* protecting health
* promoting well-being and resilience.

Health promotion teams work with groups in the community and organisations (primary health-care teams, voluntary, and statutory organisations), they identify the health needs of communities and ways of working with them to improve their health. Interventions are planned using an evidence-base working with people in a range of community settings to meet their needs. Health promotion activity can include, for example:

* physical activity
* tackling obesity
* promoting self-care for people with long-term conditions
* supporting and identifying those who are most at risk of cardiovascular disease.

Guidance has been produced that covers interventions that use a digital or mobile platform to support people to eat more healthily, become more active, stop smoking, reduce their alcohol intake, or practise safer sex. The interventions include, for example, those delivered by text message, apps, wearable devices or the internet.

Health protection teams have a responsibility to ensure that the public are protected from infectious diseases and other non-infectious hazards to health. They work with individuals, families and the wider population, which may include taking decisions on behalf of a community or population. The health protection team works with a wide range of organisations, disciplines, and agencies undertaking disease surveillance, contributing to the management of incidents, outbreaks, and control strategies, as well as leading or supporting the implementation of new directives, guidance, and policy to protect the public's health. See Figure 5.2, the 3 Ps and surveillance.

Making every contact count

Making Every Contact Count (MECC) provides an approach to behaviour change that makes use of the millions of day to day interactions that individuals and organisations have with other people in supporting them in making positive changes to their physical and mental health and well-being. MECC facilitates the opportunistic delivery of consistent and concise healthy lifestyle information, enabling individuals to participate in conversations about their health across organisations and populations.

The MECC approach is simple, it acknowledges that staff across health, local authority and voluntary sectors, have thousands of contacts on a daily with individuals and are ideally placed to promote health and healthy lifestyles. Many long-term conditions are closely linked to behavioural factors, attributable to tobacco, hypertension, alcohol, being overweight, or being physically inactive. For individuals, MECC means seeking support and taking action to improve their own lifestyle by:

* eating well
* maintaining a healthy weight
* drinking alcohol sensibly
* exercising regularly
* not smoking
* concentrating on the lifestyle issues that, when they are addressed, can make the greatest improvement in looking after their well-being and mental health.

MECC for a person's health:

* stopping smoking
* drinking alcohol only within the recommended limits
* healthy eating
* being physically active
* keeping to a healthy weight
* improving mental health and well-being.

Supporting people to make these behaviour changes has the potential to help reduce premature deaths and disability, helping achieve long-term health, social care as well as public sector savings.

The MECC approach

Adopting the MECC approach enables health and care professionals to engage people in discussions about improving their health by focusing on risk factors. Practical resources are available to support this approach including the eight steps diagram that illustrates the steps involved in scoping, planning, and implementing a MECC initiative (see Figure 5.3). MECC uses brief and very brief interventions which are delivered whenever the opportunity occurs in routine appointments and contacts. Very brief interventions take from 30 seconds to a couple of minutes. During the intervention the person is encouraged to think about change and offered help, for example, a referral or further information. A brief intervention involves a conversation, with negotiation and encouragement and can lead to referral for other interventions, or more in depth support.

Lifestyle factors

6

Ian Peate

Figure 6.1 Factors associated with lifestyle.

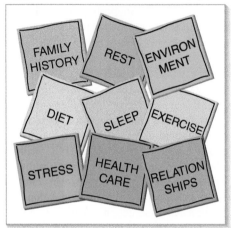

Table 6.1 Lifestyle factors impacting on health.

Factor	Impact
Smoking	Increased risk of cancer, cardiovascular disease.
Alcohol	Increased possibility of cancer.
Obesity	Cardiovascular disease, diabetes.
Illegal drug use	Risk of bloodborne viruses (HBV, HCV, HIV), mental health issues.
Sedentary lifestyles	Obesity, cardiovascular disease, cancer.
Unsafe sex	Sexually transmitted infections, unintended pregnancies.
Poor diet	Obesity, cancer, cardiovascular disease.
Stress	Hypertension, heart disease, obesity, and diabetes.

Figure 6.2 Talking about lifestyles. Source: Davey, P. et al. (Eds) (2017) Medical Ethics, Law and Communication at a Glance, p. 86, Wiley-Blackwell.

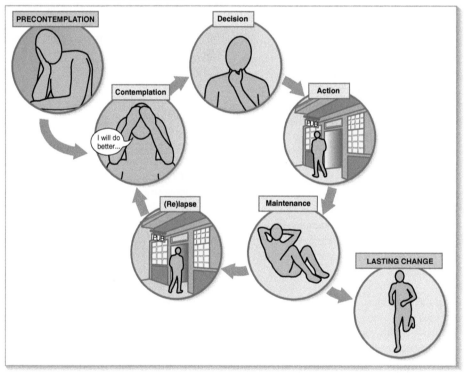

People are more than a collection of clinical data and facts, whilst clinical factors such as BMI and blood pressure can be used to evaluate health risk, there are other lifestyle factors that influence health and longevity (see Figure 6.1). This chapter is concerned with lifestyle factors and behaviour change.

Lifestyle factors

These can be seen as the adaptable behaviours and ways of life that influence a person's health and well-being. Diet, exercise, smoking, and alcohol are just some examples of lifestyle factors. Poor lifestyle choices have the real potential to result in poor

Long-term Conditions in Adults at a Glance, First Edition. Edited by Aby Mitchell, Barry Hill, and Ian Peate.

health conditions that can, in turn, impact a person's self-esteem. The impact of lifestyle can be seen in Table 6.1. People know about the harmful effects of tobacco use and obesity as well as the benefits that a balanced diet and exercise can bring. Advice provided by health-care professionals can be an important factor in helping people make decisions about lifestyle changes such as unsafe sexual activity.

A number of lifestyle factors have been recognised to play an important role in positively modifying health and their associated morbidity and mortality.

Encouraging healthier lifestyles

Many of the health issues among populations are preventable with a significant proportion resulting from unhealthy lifestyles, with poor diet, obesity, tobacco smoking, harmful alcohol consumption, and low physical activity being the biggest lifestyle contributors to ill health. There are, other causes that result in unsatisfactory health issues amongst people.

To deliver quality outcomes for patients and healthcare services, health-care professionals have to work towards ensuring that patients are informed, who have goals and a plan to improve their health. When people are motivated and ready to change an unhealthy behaviour, evidence-based techniques can be used to help them to achieve their desired outcome MECC (Making Every Contact Count) (see also Chapter 5) is an evidence-based intervention that aims to support people in making healthier choices and directing them to appropriate sources of help.

Changing behaviour and offering supporting to people to do this, for the benefit of their health can be a challenge. It is made easier when the health-care professional is knowledgeable and has an understanding of the key issues. Focusing on lifestyle changes, health promotion and education, encouraging all patients, not just those with long-term conditions should (where appropriate) be promoted.

Behavioural change

There are several theoretical behavioural change models available focusing on readiness to change and change management. It should be acknowledged that change takes time and there are number of factors that can impact change. There may be more than one consultation required before the person starts to take any action. The Transtheoretical Model of Change by Prochaska and DiClemente (also known as the Stages of Change Model), has been the basis for developing effective interventions to promote health behaviour change.

The transtheoretical model of change

The model focuses on the individual making decisions. It is a model of intentional change with the assumption that people do not change behaviours quickly and decisively, rather, change in behaviour (particularly habitual behaviour), occurs continuously through a cyclical process. People pass through a series of phases as change occurs. In Figure 6.2, the adapted seven stages are illustrated.

Pre-contemplation

At this stage people usually have no intention of changing their behaviour. They see advantages in their current behaviour or deny that they have a problem. People are often unaware that their behaviour is problematic or that it produces any negative consequences. In this stage people will often underestimate the pros of changing behaviour and they place too much emphasis on the cons of changing behaviour. Although their families, friends, neighbours, nurses, doctors, or co-workers can see the problem clearly, the typical pre-contemplator cannot. They have not yet started to think about change.

Change may occur if there is sufficient constant external pressure, however once the pressure is removed, the person will quickly revert. Those at the pre-contemplation stage are likely to avoid thinking about their problem as they feel their situation is hopeless. Acknowledging that this is a feeling that can accompany this first stage can be an effective way to motivate people. The person realises that their resistance is natural and as they work through this and all stages, they can change.

Contemplation

The person has started to think about change and has acknowledged that they have a problem and are beginning to think seriously about solving it. They recognise the dangers and risks of their current behaviour and consider the benefits as well as the downsides of changing. People in this stage may have unclear plans to make changes, often they are not ready to take any action just yet. The person will still have reasons for continuing their behaviour. Even with this recognition, the person may still feel hesitant towards changing their behaviour. People can remain in the contemplation stage for years.

Decision

The person is now preparing and making plans to change. In this stage, people are ready to take action and start to take small steps towards the behaviour change, they believe changing their behaviour can lead to a healthier life.

Action

The action stage is where people will most overtly alter their behaviour and surroundings. They stop smoking, remove all desserts from the house or they pour their last glass of wine down the drain; the person intends to keep moving forward with their behaviour change.

Maintenance

The change has been made but, support may be needed. The person is successful in avoiding former behaviours and is keeping up with new behaviours. Throughout this stage, the person has to deal with temptation so as to prevent relapse but they will become more confident that they will be able to continue their change, they are working to prevent relapse to earlier stages.

Lapse

At this stage a temporary lapse occurs and the person returns to their previous behaviour.

Relapse

Relapses are a common occurrence in any behaviour change. When a person goes through a relapse, they can experience feelings of failure, disappointment as well as frustration.

The lapse and relapse stages do not mean failure. Going through these stages demonstrate that change is difficult and expecting people to change their behaviour effortlessly, without any set back, is unreasonable. When there are setbacks, the person may require several journeys through the stages of the model to bring about lasting changes.

Socioeconomic status

Ian Peate

Table 7.1 Social class based on occupation (Registrar-General's Social Class).

Category	Description
I	Professional, etc. occupations
II	Managerial and technical occupations
III	Skilled occupations
III(N)	Non-manual
III(M)	Manual
IV	Partly skilled occupations
V	Unskilled occupations

Table 7.2 National statistics socioeconomic classification analytic classes.

Category	Description
1	Higher managerial, administrative, and professional occupations
1.1	Large employers and higher managerial and administrative occupations
1.2	Higher professional occupations
2	Lower managerial, administrative, and professional occupations
3	Intermediate occupations
4	Small employers and own account workers
5	Lower supervisory and technical occupations
6	Semi-routine occupations
7	Routine occupations
8	Never worked and long-term unemployed

Figure 7.1 An illustration of the relationship between socioeconomic group and long-term condition prevalence and severity.

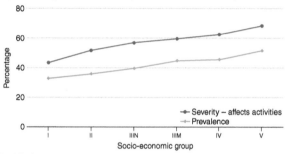

Key: I Professional, etc, occupations, II Managerial and technical occupations, III Skilled occupations, (N) Non-manual, (M) Manual, IV Partly skilled occupations, V Unskilled occupations.

Figure 7.2 Co-morbidities between the most affluent and the most deprived.
Source: Barnett et al. 2012.

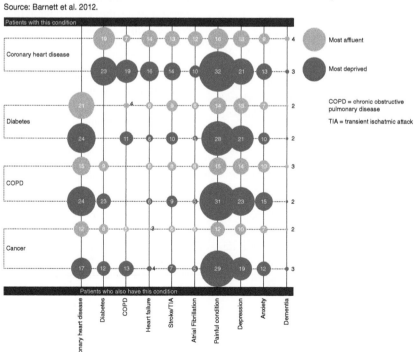

Long-term Conditions in Adults at a Glance, First Edition. Edited by Aby Mitchell, Barry Hill, and Ian Peate.
© 2023 John Wiley & Sons Ltd. Published 2023 by John Wiley & Sons Ltd.

The life chances of individuals and families are mainly determined by their position in the market and occupation is taken to be its key indicator. The occupational structure often used in socioeconomic classification is commonly used to group individuals with conceptually similar socioeconomic circumstances for the purposes of analysis. It is used as the basis of social class measures and is the focus of the stratification system.

This chapter encourages the reader to delve deeper and begin to understand the links between long-term conditions and socioeconomic deprivation so to ensure that care provision is fair and equitable.

Socioeconomic status

Socioeconomic status is a measure of an individual or family's economic and social position in relation to others, based on income, education, and occupation. There are a number of terms that are similar to socioeconomic status with many of them being used as alternatives. Social class, for example, is a construct or measure that is similar to socioeconomic status. Social class aims to situate a person's position in the social hierarchy. Measures of social class are often unidimensional unlike other systems that are finely graded on a continuous scale, limited to person's relationship to their means of production. The understanding and use of social class is not unlike the use of socioeconomic status using the terms synonymously is acceptable. The term socioeconomic position is also used synonymously. Whatever terms are used, it is important to understand that socioeconomic status is difficult to define. It is a complex and multidimensional construct that encompasses independent as well as objective characteristics such as income and education.

Socioeconomic status in the UK differs by ethnic group and gender. Indian men, for example, make up the highest proportion of people in higher managerial and professional backgrounds while women from Bangladeshi and Pakistani heritage are more likely to have never worked or be long-term unemployed.

Socioeconomic classification

All societies show some evidence of some form of hierarchy or strata. The divisions of social formations made by the hierarchy or strata is often referred to as social stratification. The socioeconomic indicators that are most commonly used to study health inequalities are:
- occupation
- income or wealth
- education.

The Registrar General's Social class system was based on the assumption that society is a graded hierarchy of occupations ranked according to skill (see Table 7.1). This system was in used from 1911–2000 in UK official statistics, individuals were assigned to a social class on the basis of their occupation or for family dependents, the occupation of the head of household.

In the UK a National Statistics Socioeconomic Classification system has replaced both the social class based on occupation system (the Registrar General's Social Class) and the socioeconomic groups system. See Table 7.2, the National Statistics Socioeconomic Classification analytic classes. There are eight main categories known as the analytic scale. The National Statistics Socioeconomic Classification measure of social class has been used in the UK since 2001 and is applied to official statistics.

The National Statistics Socioeconomic Classification is derived from occupation and employment status information. Social classifications based on occupation are used by:
- Central government to analyse social and health variation and as such direct policy and resource allocation.
- The private sector in market analysis.
- Academics in scientific analyses in health and demographic research.

Long-term conditions and socioeconomic status

Long-term conditions are more prevalent in older people and in more deprived groups. People in the poorest social class have a higher prevalence of long-term conditions (and more severity of disease) than those in the richest social class. Estimates associated with long-term conditions (the overall number of people with at least one long-term condition) suggests that the numbers are growing and the number of people with multiple long-term conditions is rising. Figure 7.1 provides an illustration of the relationship between socioeconomic group and long-term condition prevalence and severity.

Multi-morbidity is more common among deprived populations, particularly those that include a mental health problem and there is evidence suggesting that the number of conditions can be a greater determinant of a patient's use of health service resources than the specific diseases. This means that there will be a rising demand for the prevention and management of multi-morbidity as opposed to single diseases amongst the more deprived groups. Multi-morbidity among deprived populations presents a growing health-care challenge and is more common and can occur a decade earlier in those from areas of socioeconomic deprivation. By way of example, Figure 7.2 shows patterns of selected co-morbidities between those who are most affluent and the most deprived deciles.

Deprived populations are more likely to use fewer resources of all kinds available to them. This can lead to significantly poorer health outcomes and reduced quality of life and contributes to generating and maintaining inequalities. Social inequalities are created before the onset of the illness, as opposed to after it. Social inequality is the cause, not the result of or a factor in the prognosis of the illness.

Holistic needs assessment

8

Ian Peate

Figure 8.1 The whole is greater than the sum of its parts.

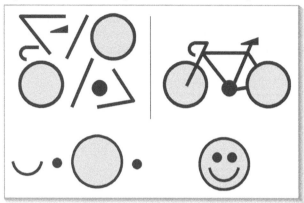

Figure 8.2 Holism and interconnectedness. Source: Bradby, M. and Oldman, C. District Nursing At A Glance, Ch. 41, pp. 92, figure 41.4, Wiley-Blackwell.

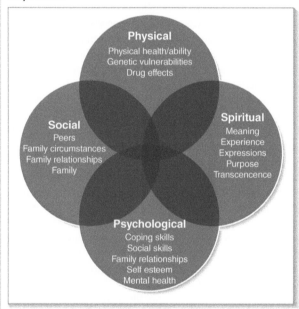

Figure 8.3 The House of Care (Licenced under the Open Government Licence v3.0).

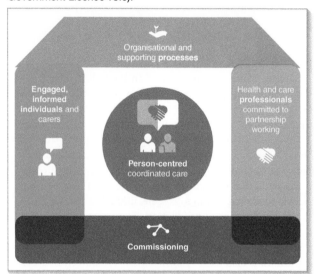

Figure 8.4 Self-management and long-term conditions.

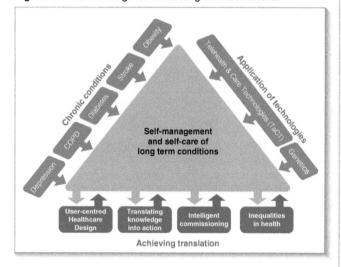

Long-term Conditions in Adults at a Glance, First Edition. Edited by Aby Mitchell, Barry Hill, and Ian Peate.
© 2023 John Wiley & Sons Ltd. Published 2023 by John Wiley & Sons Ltd.

This chapter provides an overview of holistic needs assessment in optimising care for adults with multiple long-term conditions. Needs assessments aim to improve quality of life by promoting shared decisions based on what is important to each person in terms of treatments, health priorities, lifestyle, and goals. Relationships between community groups and services have to be developed and sustained and robust evaluation systems put in place.

Holistic needs assessment

A needs assessment provides a means of ensuring that the person's concerns or problems are identified so that efforts can be made to address them. The needs assessment supports the broader aim of ensuring personalised care that reflects an individual's health and care needs, it adopts a holistic approach. The assessment should always result in a care plan or an action plan. The term 'holism' is taken from the Greek meaning all, entire or whole. The belief underpinning holism is that any given system cannot be explained by its component parts alone it is the system as a whole that determines how the parts behave (see Figure 8.1).

Holism, in health care, is a philosophy that considers the human as having physical, social, psychological, and spiritual aspects of life, all of which are closely interconnected (see Figure 8.2). A holistic assessment will take in to account all elements of a person's needs ensuring that the person is seen as a whole. When undertaking a holistic needs assessment, this should not be seen as an end in itself. It is a way of making sure that the person's concerns or problems are, in the first place identified, so efforts can then be made to address them in a systematic way. The assessment supports the broader aim of guaranteeing personalised care reflecting an individual's health and care needs. The outcome is the production of a care plan or action plan. Undertaking the assessment can impact significantly on a person's experience of their care, helping them understand that their concerns are worthy of consideration; the process provides an opportunity for discussion. It raises awareness of the sources of help they may require at that point and also what they may need at a later stage. It can also encourage people to seek help at an earlier stage than they may have done, prior to issues becoming more serious.

People have the right to be involved in discussions and make informed decisions about their care. Key to the assessment is the person who is seeking support, helping people make choices and where appropriate, to self-manage their condition on a day to day basis. This can help reduce the risk of a crisis which may culminate in an emergency or unplanned admission. Encouraging self-management will mean the health-care professional will need to signpost patients to the most appropriate resources, supporting them in making the right decision.

Those who are offered a holistic needs assessment requires nurses, doctors, and other health and care professionals to gather information from the individual as part of their treatment. During a holistic needs assessment, the person decides how much information they are willing to share about their current situation. It gives the person the opportunity for them to talk about any worries or concerns that they may have. It will help to clarify needs and ensure, if needed, appropriate referral to the relevant professionals and services.

A more consistent and systematic approach can identify those people whose needs are greatest or most immediate, allowing organisations to know where best to concentrate their efforts more effectively. A holistic needs assessment is not a one-off activity, it is carried out as a part of the diagnosis and treatment phases, forming the basis of assessment and care planning into living through their condition (survivorship) or end of life care pathways.

House of care

The House of Care is a framework for a coordinated service model. This enables patients with long-term conditions and health and care professionals to work together to establish and formulate the support required to enable patients to live well with their condition. The House of Care, a collaborative, tailored approach, uses the allegory of a house to illustrate the components that are needed to be in place to make coordinated personalised care planning a reality (see Figure 8.3).

The 'house' can be seen as a checklist to help care providers think about how they can modify their system and all its parts to improve the health and well-being of those with long-term conditions. In order to do this effectively, this requires the engagement and commitment of staff and various sectors. These include:
- National Health Service (NHS) providers
- Social care
- Public health
- Local government stakeholders.
  The 'house' acts as an enabler of care and support.
- On the right-hand wall of the 'house' is an enabled workforce is who are committed to partnership working.
- The left-hand wall, is the engaged and informed patient.
- The foundations of the 'house' are the commissioning processes and services.
- The roof covers the suitable organisational and administrative processes.
- The core of the 'house', the centre, is the patient who takes part in a collaborative care and support planning consultation (Figure 8.3).

When patients are prepared for their consultation, when they receive, informed, structured and appropriate education and emotional and psychological support, it is anticipated that they will be more able to contribute to decisions about their care.

Self-care, self-management

Those with long-term conditions, have and are, playing a central role in managing their own health, the efficacy of this is subject to their level of confidence and skill in managing tasks that can often be challenging, particularly for those with multiple conditions. People are more likely to feel confident and competent if they are encouraged and supported to engage fully in articulating their needs and capacities, agreeing on priorities, deciding goals, and jointly developing a plan for achieving these in a collaborative way. This supportive, collaborative relationship has much potential, leading to improved health outcomes. See Figure 8.4, self-management and self-care.

Holistic needs assessment is important as it identifies those people who need help, offers an opportunity for the person to think about their needs and together with health-care professionals to develop a plan about how to best meet these. It helps people to self-manage their condition, encourages teams to target support and care efforts and work more effectively by making appropriate and informed decisions.

Patient education and self-management

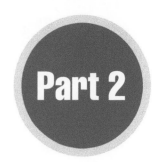

Part 2

Chapters

9   Behavioural change   22
10 Health education: developing a partnership with patients with long-term conditions   24
11 Patient responsibility   26
12 Self-care and self-management   28
13 Effectively supporting carers   30
14 Empowerment in long-term conditions   32
15 Experts by experience   34

Behavioural change

Barry Hill

Table 9.1 Motivational interviewing techniques.

Motivational interviewing techniques can be used to encourage your client to talk about change and reduce their resistance to it.

The following five techniques are advised by the Royal College of Nursing (RCN) to be easily integrated into your current approach (RCN 2022):

1. Ask open ended questions
If you use too many closed or dead-ended questions, it can feel like an interrogation. 'How often do you drink?' or 'Did you know that smoking can kill you?' Open-ended questions allow patients to tell their stories. It encourages them to do most of the talking. Your goal is to promote further dialogue so you can reflect this back to them.

Here are some examples of open-ended questions:
Tell me what has happened since we last met?
What makes you think it might be time for a change?

2. Listen reflectively
We call it reflective listening when you listen to patients then repeat or paraphrase their comments back to them. For example 'it sounds like you're not ready to quit smoking cigarettes.'
Reflections are a way of confirming what the client is feeling and communicate that you understand what they have said.
When a reflection is correct, patients will usually confirm this. If you get the reflection wrong, then this gives the client an opportunity to let you know. For example, 'No, I do want to quit, but I am worried about withdrawal symptoms and weight gain.' Your goal is to get your client to state their reasons for changing.

Here is a generic example of reflective listening:
'What I hear you saying…'
Here is a specific example of reflective listening:
'I get the sense that you are wanting to change, but you have concerns about the effect this will have on your family.'

3. Affirm/clarify
Affirmation shows that you understand and empathise with your client's struggles. It allows you to build on their strengths and past successes, improving their sense of well-being. They are best when focused on something your client has done.

Here are some examples of affirmation:
'I appreciate how hard it gets to have to hear this again.'
'You have been working hard on improving your diet.'
'I can see this is upsetting. Thanks for staying through it.'
Clarifying shows your client that you are listening and gives them an opportunity to hear what you think they said, and to respond to it. It also allows you to explain your current understanding and ask for further information if you are confused.

Here are some clarification examples:
'So, what you seem to be saying is…'
It helps to summarise and consolidate what you have discussed, so you could ask?
Who are you going to ask to support you?
What date have you decided to start?
What treatment/programme will you use?

4. Summarise
Summaries are used to relate or link what patients have already expressed and are an excellent way of expanding the discussion. To summarise effectively, you need to listen carefully to what the client is saying throughout the whole of the conversation. Also, summaries are a good way to end a conversation and can help get a particularly talkative client to move on to the next topic.

Here are some summary examples:
'It sounds like you are concerned about smoking because it is costing you a lot of money. You also said quitting will probably mean not associating with your friends any more. That doesn't sound like an easy choice.'
'Over the past three months you have been talking about exercising, and it seems that just recently you have started to recognise you are coming up with excuses for not doing it.'

5. Elicit self-motivational statements
It is your client that must have the confidence in their ability to change and not you. You can test this confidence by using scaling techniques such as the Readiness to change ruler.
If your client's readiness goes from a low number to a higher number, you can ask to follow up questions to see how they feel about the change. If the number is low, you can ask questions to explore what will make them ready.

Here are some examples of eliciting statements to support self-efficacy:
'It seems you've been working hard to quit smoking. That is different than before. How have you been able to do that?'
'Last week you weren't sure you could go a day without drinking a glass of wine, how were you able to avoid drinking for an entire past week?'

These techniques are not used in isolation but are entwined throughout the conversation. You will learn which technique to use to get the best outcome.

Many long-term conditions (LTCs) are closely linked to known behavioural risk factors. Around 40% of the UK's disability adjusted life years lost are attributable to tobacco, hypertension, alcohol, being overweight or being physically inactive. Making changes such as stopping smoking, improving diet, increasing physical activity, losing weight, and reducing alcohol

Long-term Conditions in Adults at a Glance, First Edition. Edited by Aby Mitchell, Barry Hill, and Ian Peate.
© 2023 John Wiley & Sons Ltd. Published 2023 by John Wiley & Sons Ltd.

consumption will help people reduce their risk of poor health significantly. Making every contact count (MECC) is an approach to behaviour change that utilises the millions of day to day interactions that organisations and people have with other people to encourage changes in behaviour that have a positive effect on the health and well-being of individuals, communities, and populations. Every health-care professional should use every contact with an individual to help them maintain or improve their mental and physical health and well-being; targeting the four main lifestyle risk factors: diet, physical activity, alcohol, and tobacco – whatever their speciality or the purpose of the contact. This is the basis of the Making Every Contact Count initiative in England.

The Wanless report

There is overwhelming evidence that changing people's health-related behaviour can have a major impact on some of the largest causes of mortality and morbidity. The Wanless report (Sir Derek Wanless, *Securing our Future Health* 2002 and 2006) outlined a position in the future in which levels of public engagement with health are high, and the use of preventive and primary care services are optimised, helping people to stay healthy. This 'fully engaged' scenario, identified in the report as the best option for future organisation and delivery of National Health Service (NHS) services, requires changes in behaviours and their social, economic, and environmental context to be at the heart of all disease prevention strategies. Behaviour plays an important role in people's health (for example, smoking, poor diet, lack of exercise and sexual risk-taking can cause many diseases). In addition, the evidence shows that different patterns of behaviour are deeply embedded in people's social and material circumstances, and their cultural context.

Interventions

Interventions to change behaviour have enormous potential to alter current patterns of disease. A genetic predisposition to disease is difficult to alter. Social circumstances can also be difficult to change, at least in the short to medium term. By comparison, people's behaviour – as individuals and collectively – may be easier to change. However, many attempts to do this have been unsuccessful, or only partially successful. Often, this has been because they fail to take account of the theories and principles of successful planning, delivery, and evaluation. At present, there is no strategic approach to behaviour changes across government, the NHS, or other sectors, and many different models, methods, and theories are being used in an uncoordinated way. Identifying effective approaches and strategies that benefit the population will enable public health practitioners, volunteers, and researchers to operate more effectively, and achieve more health benefits with the available resources.

Changing behaviour

Actions to bring about behavioural change may be delivered at individual, household, community, or population levels using a variety of means or techniques. The outcomes do not necessarily occur at the same level as the intervention itself. For example, population-level interventions may affect individuals, and community- and family-level interventions may affect whole populations. Significant events or transition points in people's lives present an important opportunity for intervening at some or all the levels because it is then that people often review their own behaviour and contact services. Typical transition points include leaving school, entering the workforce, becoming a parent, becoming unemployed, retirement,

and bereavement. Changing established behaviour, which has developed in response to the long-term health condition and its related problems, is a challenging task. This is evidenced by the difficulty in tackling long-term societal issues such as smoking, obesity, and alcohol misuse even when the health benefits of a 'healthy' lifestyle are compelling. Self-management is a health-care delivery model based on preventative and person-centred health systems. This new model can only be achieved through the proper use of the Intermediate Care Team (ICT), in combination with appropriate organisational changes and skills.

The role of health-care professionals

Health-care professionals working with patients can help them to build their motivation to change and support them to act when they are ready. This involves building rapport and empathy, providing support in an appropriate format, and considering the right timing. Changing behaviour should be considered as a cycle. It may start with patients being unaware of the issue, through a time when they are thinking about making a change, to when they are actively preparing to change by planning and setting goals, to when they are ready to act, and then trying to maintain the change avoiding relapse. As the stages of change need not be linear, health-care team members should start beginning to motivate their patients to change behaviours regardless. Key priorities include raising the issue and building motivation, assessing readiness to change, and supporting patients to take the next step. When using behaviour change techniques and delivering behaviour change interventions, consider the source of the intervention (who delivers it), the mode of delivery (how it is delivered) and the schedule (timing – when it is delivered).

Supporting behavioural change

There are several aspects to supporting behavioural change that will influence the outcome. These include motivational interviewing, understanding behavioural change, readiness to change, asking effective questions, interactivity – improving motivational interviewing technique and the skills used within motivational interviewing techniques (Table 9.1). Motivational interviewing (MI) is an empathetic and supportive counselling style that encourages and strengthens a client's motivation for change. Motivational interviewing techniques lead to greater participation in treatment and more positive treatment outcomes. This makes motivational interviewing an excellent tool for using with MECC. MI uses a guiding style to engage clients, clarify their strengths and aspirations, evoke their own motivations for change and promote autonomy in decision-making. MI is based on how we speak to people, which is likely to be just as important as what we say; being listened to and understood is an important part of the process of change; the person who has the problem is the person who has the answer to solving it; people only change their behaviour when they feel ready – not when they are told to do so; the solutions people find for themselves are the most enduring and effective. The four general principles of motivational interviewing are known as RULE:

Resist the urge to change the individual's course of action through didactic means. **U**nderstand it's the individual's reasons for change, not those of the practitioner, that will elicit a change in behaviour.

Listening is important; the solutions lie within the individual, not the practitioner.

Empower the individual to understand that they can change their behaviour.

10 Health education: developing a partnership with patients with long-term conditions

Pamela Arasen

Table 10.1 The barriers to effective health education can be patient-related or nurse-related.

Patient-related barriers	Nurse-related barriers
• Lack of resources such as funding due to economic situation • Lack of training materials and facilities • Limited access to learning opportunities due to age, lack of access to the Internet or an electronic device which is more frequently used for health education • Language barriers – most materials are published in the English language only • Patients with low level of literacy may be embarrassed to ask a question • Controlling family members who may make harmful decisions	• Staffing issues • Lack of planning • Time constraints – time to share valuable information • Lack of an understanding of the nurses' role in health education • A lack of awareness of the benefits of health education • Lack of nurses' training to develop knowledge, skills, and confidence to contribute in health education • Cost implications, funding issues, and employers not supporting training

Table 10.2 Using the Kirkpatrick model in diabetic patients after a health education session on self-care.

Reaction	Feedback from the patient: Measure the satisfaction of the patient with health education methods. Example: patient satisfaction after attending a session with a nutritionist on how their diet can affect their BSL
Learning	Asses to what degree the patient acquired the intended knowledge and skill – can be assessed pre and post session. Can the patient monitor their BSL?
Behaviour	Use framework and a toolkit which aim to enable and empower individual and leads them to assess and develop behaviour changes skills – is the patient complaint with their treatment pain?
Result	Post the Health Education session, the patient achieved their targeted outcomes. The BSL remain stable. Subsequent reinforcement follows.

Figure 10.1 Coaching skills in health education for patients.

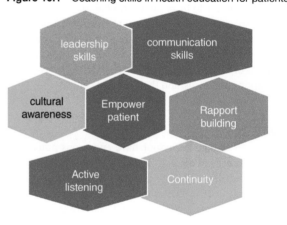

Health education and health promotion are often thought to be the same terms, but they are not interchangeable as health education is a component of health promotion. Health education is a social science with the purpose of developing individuals and uses a wide range of strategies to improve their health literacy, their knowledge about their long-term conditions, their behaviour and attitude to positively influence their self-management.

To provide holistic care, nurses who provide health education need to be aware of the five dimensions of health defined by the World Health Organization:

- physical
- mental
- emotional
- social
- spiritual.

They also need to recognise individual needs, priorities, and that people's interpretation of 'being healthy' can be different. To younger people, it could mean staying fit. To patients who have long-term conditions, which are interrelated, such as COPD, diabetes, heart failure, and depression, their needs and priorities would be different, e.g. more assistance to fulfil their activities of daily living. Therefore, their engagement with health education and their self-management may be hindered.

More importantly, health behaviours are potentially amendable when nurses have a better understanding of their role and use health education as a tool to engage the patients in health promoting behaviours.

Health education in patients with long-term conditions includes:

- Communication of information related to their long-term conditions and the primary social, economic, and environmental factors impacting on their health.
- Information on how to access services: primary, secondary, and tertiary; specialist consultation.
- Prevention strategies: providing information on individual risk factors. For example in heart failure patients, risk factors would include age, family history, past medical history.
- Risk behaviours, smoking in COPD. Heavy drinking in liver failure. Lack of compliance with treatment plan, taking medication on time, and regularly.
- Awareness that one long-term condition could lead to further complications, i.e. mental illness and higher risk of premature mortality secondary to becoming overweight and developing cardiovascular disease or type 2 diabetes.
- Nurturing motivation, skills, self-reliance, and self-efficacy through coaching sessions.

The National Society for Marketing Behaviour (2022) highlights the strengths of social marketing in health education, which includes a particular approach to achieve and sustain behavioural goals. It is therefore essential to understand patients with chronic conditions and make it easier to embrace behaviours that will improve their life quality. In health education we need to use resources that fit the patient's needs and preferences, which include but are not limited to:

- one to one patient teaching
- PowerPoint presentation
- posters
- printed materials, pamphlets
- videos from YouTube or DVDs
- group classes
- webpages such as the British Heart Foundation; COPD WebMD; Mayo Clinic.

When choosing the materials, it is pivotal to keep the patient in mind, their level of literacy and culture and whether they have access to electronic devices and the internet if they are asked to access web pages. Avoid the fear technique and inform the patient of the benefits of health education instead (see Table 10.1 barriers to effective health education).

How to use a spectrum of effective coaching skills

Health-care professionals need to develop a solid coaching relationship with their patients and the health education sessions that take place within that relationship can take a number of forms depending on the situation, i.e. the complexity of the patient's long-term condition(s) and the needs of the patients.

The nurse needs to be aware that there is a spectrum of coaching skills, and the most appropriate ones to use such as instructing, giving advice, offering guidance to be directive, i.e. in patients who have been newly diagnosed with long-term conditions. These patients may need a clearer treatment regime, advice, and guidance at this stage. On the other end, non-directive coaching skills such as reflection and active listening can be used with patients already known to their services and who are compliant with treatment plans (see Figure 10.1).

Systemic strategies to improve health education

These include:

- Using a humanistic approach to health education – treating the patients as individuals and valuing their needs and priorities.
- Creating a safe environment – to allow a climate that allows patients and their carers to talk to the health-care professionals, gain their trust, listen to one another in a non-threatening manner.
- Nurses must act as patients' advocates using their leadership, communication, and problem-solving skills to ensure patients have better access to health education, treatment, and to address any issues they may have related to health education and self-care.
- Promoting independence amongst the patients with long-term conditions and creating opportunities for the patients and their carers to take part in health education, in decision-making and in research.
- Creating Smart, Measurable, Achievable, Realistic, and Timely (SMART) goals in patients during health education sessions.
- Using strategies to address low literacy, including visual aids such as videos.
- Nurses should not assume that the patients will access the learning materials given to them. Highlight the critical importance of the information by referring to it during follow-up visits or phone calls.

For evaluating health education methods and their impact, the Kirkpatrick model is suggested. This is an internationally recognised system of appraising the results of both formal and informal training and learning programmes, grading them against four levels: reaction, learning, behaviour, and results (see Table 10.2).

Conclusion

Health education in the management of chronic illness is a critical part of any therapy as it aims at informing and empowering the patients. Specific strategies, highlighted in this chapter, can be used to target these patients to improve self-management, self-monitoring, and coping strategies with long-term conditions. Health education, including effective coaching, can improve patient outcomes through shared decision-making. Within the care team, everyone can integrate health education into their interactions.

11 Patient responsibility

Ian Peate

Figure 11.1 Deal for health and wellness.

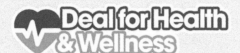
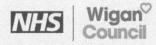

Deal for Health & Wellness — NHS | Wigan Council

Our part

Support families to give children the best start

Create training opportunities and jobs

Provide seven day access to GP services

Help communities to support each other

Help you to remain independent for as long as possible

Provide leisure facilities to help keep you healthy and active

Your part

Lead a healthy lifestyle and be a good role model

Take advantage of training and job opportunities

Register with a GP and go for regular check ups

Get involved in your community

Support older people to be independent

Make the most of leisure facilities and be active

healthwatch Wigan

5 Boroughs Partnership NHS NHS Foundation Trust

Bridgewater Community Healthcare NHS NHS Foundation Trust

Wrightington, Wigan and Leigh NHS NHS Foundation Trust

NHS Wigan Borough Clinical Commissioning Group

Box 11.1 The seven key principles that guide the NHS in all that it does. Source: NHS Constitution 2021.

1 The NHS provides a comprehensive service, available to all.
2 Access to NHS services is based on clinical need, not an individual's ability to pay.
3 The NHS aspires to the highest standards of excellence and professionalism.
4 The patient will be at the heart of everything the NHS does.
5 The NHS works across organisational boundaries.
6 The NHS is committed to providing best value for taxpayers' money.
7 The NHS is accountable to the public, communities, and patients that it serves.

Long-term Conditions in Adults at a Glance, First Edition. Edited by Aby Mitchell, Barry Hill, and Ian Peate.
© 2023 John Wiley & Sons Ltd. Published 2023 by John Wiley & Sons Ltd.

The NHS belongs to all of us. It is there to improve our health and well-being, supporting us to keep mentally and physically well, to get better when we are ill and when we are unable to fully recover, to stay as well as we can to the end of our lives. There are things we can all do for ourselves and for one another so as to help the National Health Service (NHS) work more effectively and to ensure that the resources are used responsibly (Figure 11.1).

The NHS Constitution

The NHS Constitution for England outlines the principles and values of the NHS in England. It sets out rights to which patients, public as well as staff are entitled and promises which the NHS is committed to achieve, together with responsibilities, which the public, patients, and staff owe to each other to ensure that the NHS can operate in a fair and effective way.

The NHS Constitution is accompanied by the Handbook to the NHS Constitution, this sets out current guidance on the rights, pledges, duties, and responsibilities established by the Constitution, the Constitution has to be renewed every 10 years and the Handbook at least every 3 years. These requirements for renewal are legally binding. They guarantee that the principles and values underpinning the NHS are subject to regular review and re-commitment; and that any government which seeks to alter the principles or values of the NHS, or the rights, pledges, duties, and responsibilities set out in this Constitution, have a obligation to engage in a full and transparent discussion with the public, patients, and staff. There are seven key actions that guide the NHS in what it does recognise you can make a significant contribution to your own and your family's good health.

- Register with a GP practice.
- Treat NHS staff and other patients with respect.
- Provide accurate information about your health, condition and status.
- Keep appointments or cancel within reasonable time.
- Follow the course of treatment which you have agreed.
- Participate in important public health programmes such as vaccination.
- Ensure those closest to you are aware of your wishes about organ donation.
- Give feedback, both positive and negative, about treatment and care received.

Shared responsibilities

Good quality health care is shared responsibility. Engaging in discussion, asking questions, seeking information and exploring alternatives improves communication and understanding of a person's health and treatment (see also Chapter 9). The care that patients receive can depend, in part, on the patient's active participation. Sharing responsibilities can help health and care providers promote the safe and appropriate delivery of care.

There should be a greater emphasis on shared responsibilities between health care professionals and patients so that improvements can occur in the provision of health and care. The NHS Constitution highlights the seven key principles that guide the NHS (see Box 11.1). In order for shared responsibility to work in an effective way this will require health care professionals to adopt different working practices so that patients and the public can become more involved in decisions that are being made regarding their health and well-being.

It is acknowledged that most people are already taking responsibility for their health and care, however there could be more done to reduce excessive reliance on health and care services and to make the use of people's own expertise. People should be supported in making healthy choices with an emphasis on shared decision-making a reality: there should be no decision about me, without me. The aspiration for patients and clinicians to come together and arrive at decisions about treatment together, with a shared understanding of the person's condition, the available options and the risks and benefits of each of those can become a reality. The patient is the most important primary care provider.

Shared decision-making supports the patients' own preferences being considered and can lead to more conservative treatment decisions being made than when health and care professionals do not involve patients. This consideration is important particularly in view of growing evidence of overdiagnosis and overtreatment, this seeks to improve conversations between patients and clinicians, in order to avoid 'too much medicine'.

The underpinning reason for shared responsibility results from the changing disease burden. Advances in medicine have resulted in reductions in premature deaths that had arisen from major killers, for example, heart disease, stroke, and cancers. As well as an increase in numbers of those who are living with at least one long-term condition, including diabetes, chronic respiratory diseases and heart failure. Caring for people with these conditions makes up the bulk of the need and demand in society and this requires care providers to offer a different response. The prevalence of lifestyle-induced diseases is increasing globally and non-communicable diseases are overtaking infectious diseases as the leading cause of morbidity and mortality.

The primary purpose of the health-care system was, largely, to provide intermittent treatment intervention for those with acute illnesses, it now needs to provide joined-up support for older people and others who are living with long-term conditions. Contemporary health-care systems must also provide ongoing care for the increasing numbers of people who have survived cancers and other major causes of premature death due to the advances in medicine, action plans, and commissioning of services which need to reflect this as they make their response.

Prevention and treatment relies on people playing their part in making healthy choices, for example in relation to rising levels of overweight and obesity, substance dependency in the population and preventing or delaying the onset and progression of chronic diseases, such as chronic obstructive pulmonary disease (COPD), cancer, and diabetes.

The public see themselves as responsible for working with health professionals to make healthy choices and use services appropriately. Responsibility is a shared responsibility between patients and the public on the one hand and health professionals on the other. It is the relationship between the various parties that is the real meaning of health care, the interaction between a proactive health and care team and an informed, empowered patient and family.

Self-care and self-management

12

Barry Hill

Table 12.1 Self-management.

Self-management is what a person with a long-term health condition does every day. This may include:
• recognising and dealing with symptoms (monitoring a condition)
• taking medication(s)
• managing other treatments
• attending various appointments
• making lifestyle changes
• coping with the emotional effects of the condition.
To do this well a person needs to have the right information, education, support, and services. Learning how to manage their condition may help them feel better, stay active and live well.

Table 12.2 Some examples of self-management support.

Self-management support aims to increase a person's knowledge, confidence, and skills when looking after their health. Self-management support is about helping people to
• learn more about their condition
• set goals, problem solve, and make plans to live a healthier life.
Self-management support is not a one-off, but is an on-going part of the care of a long-term health condition.

There are many different types of self-management support. Some examples include:
• Regular reviews by different members of the health-care team.
• Information about the long-term condition.
• Action plans, for use when symptoms get worse, e.g. asthma action plan or COPD communication plan.
• Group-based education programmes and workshops.
• Cardiac rehabilitation for people with heart conditions.
• Pulmonary rehabilitation for people with Asthma or COPD.
• Lifestyle change supports. Examples include stop smoking services or supports to increase physical activity levels.
• Support with dealing with the emotional aspects of long-term health conditions for example counselling.
• Support groups such as Cardiac Support Groups, Diabetes Support Groups, and COPD support groups.
• Social Prescribing or Health and well-being community referral.
• Chronic disease self-management programmes such as the HSE Living Well programme.

Long-term Conditions in Adults at a Glance, First Edition. Edited by Aby Mitchell, Barry Hill, and Ian Peate.
© 2023 John Wiley & Sons Ltd. Published 2023 by John Wiley & Sons Ltd.

Long-term conditions

Millions of people in the UK are living with long-term conditions. A long-term health condition is one which can be treated and managed but usually not cured. Examples include asthma, chronic obstructive pulmonary disease (COPD), diabetes mellitus, heart conditions, and stroke. Having a long-term health condition usually brings change to a person's life. People with long-term health conditions have an important role in their own health care. Family members or carers may also have a role to play. It is important that people have a full understanding of their condition. They need to know how to manage it and how it will affect their life.

Up to a quarter of those affected have more severe symptoms and are at higher risk of hospital admission. Most, however, are leading full and active lives with only occasional contact with health professionals and provide much of their care themselves, altering drug doses and adapting their lifestyles in response to subtle changes in symptoms. These decisions and behaviours constitute 'self-management' of long-term conditions and affect a patient's overall health and well-being significantly (Table 12.1). The role of health professionals in ensuring that patients understand their condition and supporting them to self-manage it is essential (Table 12.2). Government policy on long-term conditions identifies support for self-management as one of three key approaches to improving services and maintaining good health. There is evidence that effective self-management can reduce hospitalisation and accident and emergency attendances.

Living with a long-term condition brings challenges and it's important to have the confidence, support, and information to manage health. Self-care can help patients make the most of living with their health condition/s, rather than avoiding or missing out on things because of it. Self-care puts the patient in control of their care which is supported and enhanced by health-care professionals when required. Research shows that people with long-term conditions who take more control of their health feel more able to cope with their health problem, have better pain management, fewer flare ups, and more energy. It is more important to emphasise the importance of taking individual accountability for health. This includes responsibilities such as adopting a healthier lifestyle, staying active, eating healthily, only using alcohol in moderation and not smoking.

Self-care

Self-care is integral to the governments approach to personalisation, enabling people to be at the heart of decision-making about what matters to them. The personalisation agenda can engender resilience and self-care through social prescribing – which is a means of enabling any health-care professional to refer patients for support either to a link worker – to provide them with a face to face conversation during which they can learn about the possibilities and design their own personalised care, or even to wider networks for example to leisure centres, or specific programmes such as exercise, arts, gardening, to name but a few to support people to do things to support their wider well-being.

Social prescribing

Social prescribing has been referred to as several things; community referral or asset-based, person-centred approaches, there is no agreed single term used to describe social prescribing. It is, however, a key method to support asset-based person-centred self-care. Collectively, the UK personalisation agenda, using socially prescribed services such as 'arts on prescription', gardening, or exercise, utilises an individual's strengths to enable them to manage their own conditions. At an even more fundamental level these things help people get out, they reduce social isolation and improve community networks. Find out more about social prescribing.

Personal responsibility and accountability for health

Self-care starts with an individual taking responsibility for making daily choices about their lifestyle, such as brushing their teeth, eating healthily, or choosing to exercise. At the opposite end of the continuum is major trauma where responsibility for care is entirely in the hands of the health-care professionals, until the start of recovery when self-care can begin again. The National Health Service (NHS) can support people to self-care at any point during the continuum. The reality is that probably around 80% of all care in the UK is self-care, from people managing their own minor illness and longer-term chronic conditions and generally how they take care of themselves.

Self-care and self-management

Many people use the terms self-care and self-management interchangeably. However, there are important distinctions between the two. Self-management will usually be used in relation to long-term, chronic health conditions while self-care applies to acute illness or injuries. Self-management is about coping with long-term health conditions and managing the emotional and practical issues they present. Self-care focuses more on treatment. Around 15 million people in England have one or more long-term conditions, and this is predicted to rise by a third over the next ten years. Self-management is the systematic process of learning and practising skills which enable individuals to manage their health condition on a day-to-day basis, through practising and adopting specific behaviours which are central to managing their condition, making informed decisions about care, and engaging in healthy behaviours to reduce the physical and emotional impact of their illness, with or without the collaboration of the health-care system. This means that self-management offers a way for people with long-term conditions to create a more sustainable way of living with a health condition. As a health-care professional people have a duty of care to support patients in making healthy choices and in directing people to useful sources of information. This includes the provision of advice, education, and training to help people manage their condition, to know when to seek medical help and when they can self-manage their symptoms.

Effectively supporting carers

Rachael Betty

Figure 13.1 Examples of different types of support.

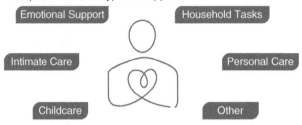

Emotional Support	Household Tasks	Intimate Care	Personal Care	Childcare	Other
Monitoring	Shopping, cooking	Washing	Giving medications	Caring for children	Paying bills
Offering hope	Cleaning, laundry	Dressing	Changing dressings	Leading on school links	Advocacy
Maintaining safety	Life admin; advocacy	Supporting toilet use	Mobility assistance	Ad hoc and planned	Translating

Figure 13.2 Carer well-being model; factors affecting well-being.
Source: Heath, A., Carey, L.B. and Chong, S (2018) Helping Carers Care: An Exploratory Study of Factors Impacting Informal Family Carers and Their Use of Aged Care Services. Journal of Religion and Health 57:1146–1167.

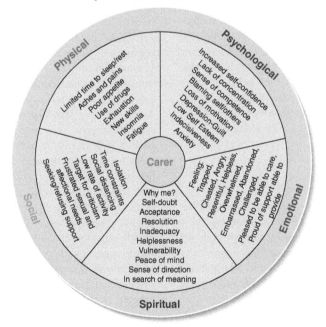

1 in 8 adults across the UK are carers; every day another 6000 people become carers, and 600 people leave work due to their carer responsibilities. Approximately 5 million people – 1/7th of the workforce – are juggling work alongside caring responsibilities, and over a million carers support more than one person – saving the economy an annual £132 billion. This excludes those who do not see themselves as carers; it takes an average of two years for people to begin to acknowledge their carer role.

Who are carers?

Carers are defined as anyone who looks after a family member, partner, or friend who needs help due to an illness, frailty, disability, mental health problem or addiction and cannot cope without their support. The physical and emotional nature of the role will vary widely as outlined in Figure 13.1. People requiring care may not recognise the support that others around them provide; due to perceiving more independence, associated stigma, feeling infantilised, or difficulty perceiving others' needs due to the pervasive nature of their own needs. These factors can make it more difficult for carers to be easily identified; and therefore may require the use of different terminology and creative communication to ensure carers are acknowledged and met.

Signs of 'burnout'

Caregiver 'burnout' is well-documented, particularly among people caring for older people with dementia as they account for 50% of carers; signs include uncharacteristic lack of compassion and irritability, not wanting to be around their loved ones, neglecting their own needs, resentment, and increased use of maladaptive coping strategies. While carers are encouraged to take a break and share their caring responsibilities, many may feel unable to do so or unsure of how to do so if they are not receiving any carer support. A total of 72% of carers experienced mental ill health and 61% physical health issues as a result of their caring role; reporting common themes of loneliness or social isolation – and a carers' risk of suicide is three times the national average.

It is clear that the cost of not 'caring for carers' is far more devastating than the potential economic impact.

What is the emotional impact of caring?

Carers report experiencing grief from the loss of their loved ones with dementia while they are still alive; particularly common in chronic or degenerative conditions where there are pre-morbid personality changes. When the person with dementia does pass away, carers may experience further grief, a lack of purpose, a reduction in social support or a sense of relief; which can add to the shame and guilt that carers often experience and can feel 'taboo' to discuss openly.

Carers may also fear judgment from others about care quality. Shame, guilt, and blaming themselves or others for their loved ones' illness and ruminating on what could have been different can create difficulty in recognising progress, reluctance to access support or feelings of 'weakness' for requiring support. Despite this, connection with others in similar situations consistently reduces isolation; see Figure 13.2.

Given the variety of valid emotions experienced by carers across their journey, practitioners should be mindful of the language they use when supporting carers to avoid the expectation of a particular emotional response and allow them to express their thoughts and feelings without judgment. It is difficult for carers to be open about concerns where they perceive an emotional expectation; 'how do you feel about your relative coming home?' is far more likely to generate an honest response than, 'isn't it great that they are being discharged?'

How to effectively support carers

What carers want is recognition and respect, information sharing, signposting, flexible, and patient-centred care, whole family consideration, recognition of own needs as well as carer needs, and to be treated with dignity and compassion. Tokenistic attempts at carer involvement, such as seeing a 'getting to know you' documentation as a one-off exercise, or consultation after a clinical decision has been made can feel more alienating and frustrating than no contact at all; the 'triangle of care' model (available online via NHS England, 2023) demonstrates an equal partnership between service users, carers, and practitioners to maximise recovery and well-being.

Consent to share remains consistently cited as a barrier to support from services. While patient confidentiality is paramount, carers usually want to share information rather than receive it. Practitioners should feel confident in discussing general information with carers, and should not use this as a reason to avoid responding unless there are clear safeguarding issues. Systemic complexities can also make it difficult to access services; when multiple agencies feel a different service is more appropriate, but expect the carer to advocate and liaise rather than clarifying this with the other agency and requesting they make direct contact. Trust and mutual respect are built through being human; listening, offering validation and explanation, and consistency – which needs to be systemically embedded as well as individually.

Conclusion and summary

Carers' needs can best be met through respect and acknowledgement of the importance of the role they play in recovery. They should feel able to question clinical decision-making – especially when those decisions involve expectations on their time and resources. Familiarity with best practices, legal requirements, the National Health Service (NHS)'s long-term commitment to carers and sound knowledge of what is available both locally and nationally to support carers is vital to ensure signposting, ongoing support, and advocacy are routinely shared with those in a caring role.

While challenging, being a carer can also be an incredibly rewarding and valuable experience, leading to stronger relationships, knowledge, and mutual understanding. Many carers go on to support others in similar situations to themselves or their loved ones. Balancing validation of the realities of the current situation while maintaining hope for recovery and the future is both dynamic and delicate, and requires significant interpersonal skills, empathy, and human connection, but is essential in promoting lasting recovery.

14 Empowerment in long-term conditions

Sara Tavares

Figure 14.1 Patient health-related outcomes resulting from patient empowerment.

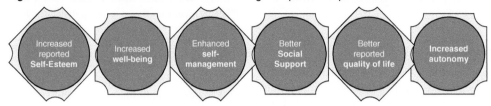

Figure 14.2 Key contributions to active participation.

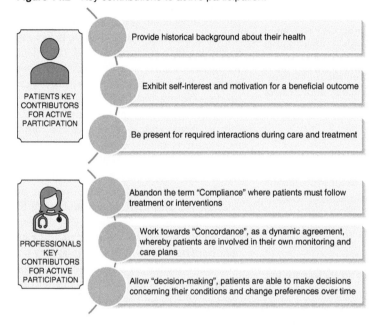

Figure 14.3 Self-management stages and indicators of empowerment.

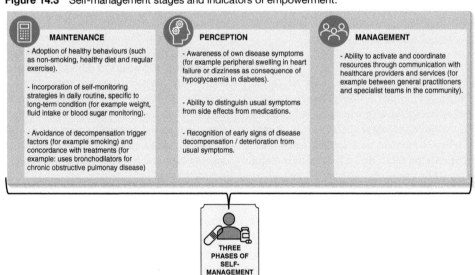

Long-term Conditions in Adults at a Glance, First Edition. Edited by Aby Mitchell, Barry Hill, and Ian Peate.
© 2023 John Wiley & Sons Ltd. Published 2023 by John Wiley & Sons Ltd.

Trends in health care reflect an increasingly complex ageing population with multiple long-term conditions without curative options, but for which disease trajectory, progression or symptomatic burden can be often haltered through medication regimes or other evidence-based interventions. Desired health-related outcomes from these interventions are usually translated into lower mortality, morbidity, and (re)hospitalisation rates, leading to enhanced quality of life. To achieve these, chronic patients are asked to interact with health-care professionals with patient participation and engagement being a fundamental aspect of sustainable health policies focusing on long-term/chronic conditions. As an illustration of this relevance, the National Health System (NHS) identifies in its recent long-term plan, the urgency to facilitate change in patient's roles towards self-care, prevention, and personalisation of care, shifting from traditional paternalistic health care to contemporaneous patient-centred approaches.

Definition of empowerment

Achieving active participation in clinical practice faces well-known barriers such as time constrains, lack of resources, and professionals training. To address these problems and improve patient participation, from a policy perspective, the concept of empowerment emerged with view to increase autonomy, power, and influence of individuals and communities. Empowerment is a multi-level and multi-dimensional construct including individual, psychological, community, and organisational processes.

In health-care patient empowerment is a core value of patient-centred approaches, and although no consensual definition is found in the literature, it can be described as patients' capacity, knowledge, power, and ability to control and manage their own illness, as well as the ability to be more involved in their care and shared-decision-making. Patients' discussions regarding their treatment options are nowadays both an ethical and legal requirement. Following the Montgomery vs. Lanarkshire Health Board case, patients are legally required to be fully informed of their condition and all possible associated risks to be able to provide informed consent. This translates in exercising the ethical principal of autonomy, whereby patients are given enough information to be able to decisions, weighting the risks in relation to perceived benefits. However, empowerment goes beyond informed decisions and consent, as empowered individuals are not only engaged, motivated, and actively involved in care, but also have the knowledge, skills, and health literacy confidence to self-manage their conditions (Figure 14.1).

Fundamental components of the empowerment process

When discussing empowerment and patient-centred approaches, a wide-range of similarly overlapping concepts are often described and used interchangeably, however these all have slightly different meanings since empowerment is a concept, a process and a result. The following constitute essential components to patient empowerment.

Active and personalised patient participation

A series of interactions between patients and health-care systems are required to efficiently manage long-term conditions. These interactions must follow a transactional communication approach, offering the opportunity for patients to be involved in their care by aiding to the diagnosis process and sharing personal preferences and priorities towards management plans. An active and personalised participation requires equal contribution from both patients and health-care professionals as shown in Figure 14.2.

Patient knowledge, education, and health literacy

On each interaction, providing patients with personalised and tailored information, abandoning jargon and patronising tones is essential to a successful educational process. This partnership must allow sufficient time to enhance patients' understanding on own disease physiology, trajectory, symptoms, and early signs of deterioration. Polypharmacy is usually present in long-term conditions; therefore, medication regimes must be explained to a level where patients are able to distinguish side-effects from treatments to those expected from their own medical condition, creating a safe and personalised care plan according to specific disease and medication regime.

Communicating information is only the first step in this educational process, as patients need to develop health literacy, when they are able to interpret information, to make informed decisions about their health care. Patients' refusal to accept recommendations, procedures, or interventions based on their personal views is a common situation in clinical practice, posing as a dual moral and ethical challenge, especially when individuals have been deemed as capable to make informed and autonomous decisions. Whereas patients have the right to autonomy, professionals have the legal and regulated duty to promote well-being and advocate towards beneficence (do good). The ideal empowerment strategy in promoting health literacy, avoids manipulative strategies using persuasion techniques where patients are led to adopt interventions that suit healthcare professionals' views, and works towards tackling lack of knowledge, bad habits, or bias through education. The process of introducing a choice, describing the options and helping patients to explore their preferences, resulting in a decision defines the concept of shared decision making.

Self-efficacy or personal control

Once health literacy is promoted and tailored education provided, patients must believe they have the capabilities to produce change and reach a goal in the context of their disease. When achieved, these individuals display higher motivation than those with low self-efficacy and feel in control of their conditions even when not in contact with healthcare professionals. As a healthcare professional it is important to recognise mood, emotional states, physical reaction, and stress might have an influence on patients' ability and perception of self-efficacy can vary according to disease trajectory (for example decompensating stages of a chronic condition might lead to patients feel they have lost temporary control).

Self-management skills

Self-management or self-care are often used interchangeably, but the latter is a broader term that goes beyond healthy lifestyle behaviours. In conjunction with family, community, and healthcare system, optimal self-management occurs in three interlinked phases as illustrated in Figure 14.3. It is an iterative process whereby patients use disease specific knowledge, personal control, and health literacy to recognise a change, decide to implement a treatment strategy, being then able to evaluate response and maintain quality of life. It is important to allow patients time to process, grieve and adjust to new ways of life. Empowerment cannot be reduced to a simple method of active participation or self-management but as a multi-dimensional process that occurs as result of effective interactions between individuals and the healthcare system.

Experts by experience

Sue Tiplady

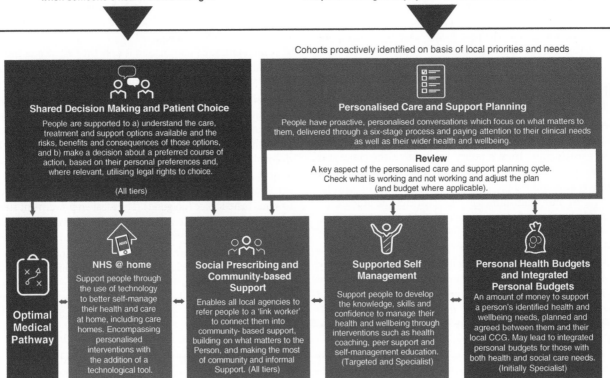

Figure 15.1 Person-centred care model (NHS England 2021). Available at: https://www.england.nhs.uk/wp-content/uploads/2018/10/personalised-care-operating-model-2021.pdf.

Experts by experience

The importance of involving people in their own health and social care has been a source of discussion for decades. Government policy places a legal duty within Health and Social Care to ensure that patients and their carer representatives must be involved in all aspects of their care and promote shared decision-making with the principles of 'no decision about me without me' (Health and Social Care Act 2012). There are many labels being applied interchangeably to people and are usually related to a level of involvement with their own care, the development delivery and evaluation of service provision, research, and education these include service users, and experts by experience. Experts by Experience (EbE) are people with experience of using services as either a service user or a carer who are interested in undertaking activities with health and social care programmes and within health and social care services. EbEs provide a valuable part of helping organisations to ensure that they develop their services in relation to the needs of service users and carers. Essentially, these involvement opportunities are designed to provide an opportunity for people with a lived experience to participate in service development while gaining skills or experience as they move forward on their recovery journey. It is worth noting that whilst there may some commonality with other people living with the same or similar condition, they are an expert with their own personal experiences.

The role of EbEs in LTC

The NHS Long-Term Plan acknowledged that despite the move towards people having more choice and control regarding their own care that there was still more work required to work with patients as partners in envisioning person-centred care. People who are living with their long-term conditions should be working in partnership as equals with the health and social care practitioners that they have contact with. It is vital that practitioners appreciate the person is an expert in their own care and understand 'what matters to them' rather than 'what is the matter with someone'; this is crucial for effective care and support planning. In addition to being an expert in their own care, EbEs are often involved in either assisting others in understanding a condition or more widely in aiding organisations develop services which meet the needs of service users. The core skills that are needed for this role generally include:
• The ability to talk about 'lived' experience in an open and honest way.
• The ability to support others when they talk about themselves and their experiences.
• The ability to get on with others in a friendly way. This is an excellent skill to have and one that will be used more than any other. Very often EbEs work together as a group.
• Finally, having an interest in helping to improve health care, and what organisations do for people living with long-term conditions.

EbEs in education

Within professional standards it has been identified that health and social care education must involves service users in the development and delivery of programmes of study. The pedagogical value of service user involvement in education is evident and extremely positive. Research evaluations into holistic health including students has been applauded and evaluated as inspirational. Research into social work showed that there are several benefits, including enhanced awareness of the lived experience; taking on board suggestions of good practice from service user and carers; developing a more critical 'real life' understanding; and a culture of recognising service users and carers as experts. It has been suggested that involvement of service users in health-care education can facilitate the development of people's caring skills by promoting understanding of the reality of service users' situations.

EbEs in clinical practice

Individuals living with a long-term condition are best placed to understand the effect and impact of the condition for them and their carers and families. Active involvement of people in their own care and treatment is key if person-centred care is to be achieved. Shared decision-making is a process in which people who experience a change in their health work together with clinicians to select tests, treatments, management, or support packages. This is based on the best available evidence and the individual's informed preferences. More specifically, shared decision-making is a conversation, or series of conversations, that should include evidence-based information about all reasonable options (Figure 15.1).

EbEs in research and audit

The Care Quality Commission (CQC) duty is to regulate health and adult social care in England. As part of the inspection process EbEs are a crucial part of the assessment process and using their experience they speak to service users and staff they will observe how services are being delivered, their input is valuable in assessing how well care standards are being achieved. In 2020 the Care Quality Commission (CQC) awarded the contract to deliver Experts by Experience services across England to the national charity 'Choice Support'. The CQC identify an EbE as a person who has had a recent personal experience within the last five years of using or caring for someone who uses physical health, mental health, and or social care services. An example of how CQC reports can help people living with a long-term condition can be seen in the example My Diabetes My Care (2016); this highlighted views of the 'lived experience' of areas of good practice and identified areas where improvements could be made. Within research, the Health Research Authority (HRA) identify that involving people with relevant lived experience in research can improve the quality and relevance of studies. Experts by Experience can also become peer researchers; peer research can give a voice to those with relevant perspectives and experiences to share their views with researchers who understand 'the lived experience' putting them in ideal position to engage others living with long-term conditions.

Long-term conditions

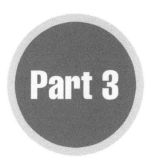

Part 3

Chapters

16 Alcohol dependency 38
17 Anorexia nervosa 40
18 Arthritis 42
19 Asthma 44
20 Angina 46
21 Anxiety 48
22 Atrial fibrillation 50
23 Bipolar affective disorder 52
24 Bulimia nervosa 54
25 Bronchiectasis 56
26 Cancer 58
27 Chronic fatigue syndrome 60
28 Chronic venous insufficiency 62
29 Chronic obstructive pulmonary disease (COPD) 66
30 Coronary artery Disease 68
31 Chronic liver disease 70
32 Depression 72
33 Diabetes mellitus type 1 74
34 Diabetes mellitus type 2 78
35 Dual diagnosis 82
36 Diverticular disease 84
37 Epilepsy 88
38 Heart failure 90
39 HIV 92
40 Hypertension 94
41 Inflammatory bowel disease 96
42 Multiple sclerosis 98
43 Parkinson's disease 100
44 Peripheral arterial disease 102
45 Psoriasis 104
46 Rheumatoid arthritis 106
47 Sickle cell 108
48 Schizophrenia 110
49 Vascular dementia 112
50 Viral hepatitis 114
51 Visual impairment 116

16 Alcohol dependency

Leticia Wedderburn and Helen Phillips

Figure 16.1 Alcohol unit reference.

This is one unit of alcohol...

 Half pint of regular lager or cider

 1 small glass of wine

 1 single measure of spirits

 1 small glass of sherry

 1 single measure of aperitif

...and each of these is more than one unit

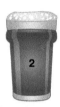 **2** Pint of regular beer, lager or cider

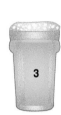 **3** Pint of premium beer, larger or cider

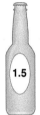 **1.5** Alcopop or can/bottle of regular lager

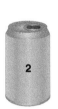 **2** Can of premium lager or strong lager

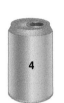 **4** Can of super strong lager

 2 Glass of wine (175 ml)

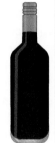 Bottle of wine

Long-term Conditions in Adults at a Glance, First Edition. Edited by Aby Mitchell, Barry Hill, and Ian Peate.
© 2023 John Wiley & Sons Ltd. Published 2023 by John Wiley & Sons Ltd.

Alcoholism is the most severe type of alcohol addiction and is characterised by an inability to control drinking patterns. Alcohol use disorder (AUD) refers to alcohol addiction or alcoholism when diagnosed. On the same note, AUD is a pattern of alcohol use marked by an inability to manage to drink, obsession with alcohol, or continued use of alcohol despite issues. This long-term condition also results in the user requiring more alcohol to have the same effects and to prevent withdrawal symptoms. It is accepted that any degree of drinking that occasionally tends to spiral out of control is a component of alcohol consumption disorder. People who struggle with alcoholism frequently believe they cannot operate adequately without alcohol. This can have a wide range of negative effects on their personal life, career objectives, interpersonal connections, and health. Consistent alcohol misuse has substantial negative effects that might deteriorate over time and lead to health complications.

Prevalence

There were 814 595 alcohol-related hospital admissions in England between 2020 and 2021. The Health Survey for England, 2021, states that 1 in 4 people use alcohol excessively. Alcohol-related accidents, chronic and acute illness, and hospital admissions may occur from or be influenced by this. Consequently, it is recommended that straightforward alcohol advice is provided as it has been proven to reduce a person's weekly drinking up to 34% (8.7 fewer units per week), which has a considerable impact on health risks. Health advice can lead to 1 in 8 adults reducing their alcohol intake. Adults are twice as likely to limit their drinking six to twelve months following professional intervention.

Screening

Alcohol harm identification test (AUDIT)

The World Health Organization (WHO) developed a comprehensive 10-question AUDIT (Gov.UK 2022) (see Figure 16.1). This technique identifies problems with alcohol consumption. AUDIT examines question such as: *'How frequently do you consume alcoholic beverages?' 'On an average day that you drink alcohol, how many units do you consume?' 'How many times in the last year were you so drunk that you couldn't recall what occurred the night before?'*. The individual's replies are scored from 0 to 4 points, with a score of 0 to 7 points denoting minimal risk and 8 to 15 points denoting danger. Additionally, a score of 16–19 indicates increased risk, and a score of more than 20 indicates potential dependency. The medical professional must make a referral to a specialist in alcohol harm assessment especially when the score more than 20 points.

The alcohol identification and brief advice (alcohol IBA)

The Alcohol IBA screening method is another option. It enables professionals to identify people whose drinking may have a negative impact on their health, currently or in the future, and to provide straightforward, structured advice aimed at lowering that risk. The strategy was created in conjunction with NICE Public Health Guideline PH24 and Public Health England. The recommendation addresses alcohol-related issues and seeks to avoid and identify such issues as early as feasible by combining policy and practice. As a common component of practice, healthcare practitioners should identify alcohol risk factors and offer succinct recommendations (Public Health England 2017). All hospital settings provide chances to 'Make Every Contact Count', thus it is critical that personnel have the most recent knowledge to communicate with patients about the effects that lifestyle choices have on their health. IBA is the providing of 'simple short advice' after determining how much the patient drinks and any potential difficulties they may be having. IBA has proven to be beneficial in assisting people in lowering their risk of alcohol-related illness and can also be provided by non-alcohol experts.

Symptoms

Any alcohol consumption that endangers a person's health or safety or results in alcohol-related issues is considered unhealthy. The warning signals of alcohol misuse might sometimes be obvious and other times take longer to manifest. The likelihood of a full recovery increases dramatically when alcoholism is identified in its early stages. Unable to manage alcohol use, wanting alcohol even while sober, and prioritising alcohol above personal duties are all typical indications of alcoholism. AUD is of concern particularly when a person is deemed to be drinking alcohol frequently and in unsafe circumstances, such as when driving or swimming, as well as failing to engage in life activities, such as working or studying. Alcohol excess can lead to an altered consciousness, resulting in a coma or brain damage. Alcohol consumption generally results in various difficulties such as liver disease, digestive issues, cardiac issues, complications from diabetes, and may cause foetal abnormalities. It is also recognised to cause mental health problems and challenging behaviour.

Treatment approach

There are several treatment options available to people who are alcohol dependent. Although each patient's treatment plan is unique, the normal course of therapy consists of detoxification, rehabilitation, and maintenance. Detoxification is the first step in alcohol addiction rehabilitation, and it should be carried out with the assistance of clinical specialists owing to the possibility of severe and painful withdrawal symptoms (NICE 2019). This is because people frequently receive medications to manage the unpleasant withdrawal side-effects. The second stage is rehabilitation, which entails rigorous treatment regimens and necessitates that the inpatient person checks into a facility for a predetermined amount of time, often 30, 60, or 90 days. Individuals might enrol in a rehabilitation programme through outpatient treatment while carrying on with their daily activities. The healing process does not complete after rehabilitation is complete. Long-term sobriety necessitates regular therapy and may involve recovery tools including support groups and counselling. These will increase the probability of sobriety.

Anorexia nervosa

Tichaona Mubaira

Lived experience perspective

I suffered from the age of 12 until I finally sought help at the age of 24. At that point, I was pretty desperate and hopeless. I thought that change would never ever be possible and therapy was such hard work. It took a long time but I eventually entered recovery and have never looked back. My life now is wonderful – and I never thought that possible.

Anorexia sufferer

Table 17.1 Eating disorder and anorexia.

Eating disorder in general	Anorexia nervosa specifically
• 1.25–3.4 million people affected in the UK • 25% of those affected are male • Most commonly develop during adolescence • Most common in ages 16–40 yrs • More likely to develop if there is family history • Highest mortality rates among psychiatric disorders • Better chances of recovery if appropriate treatment initiated earlier • Equal distribution across social classes	• Around 10% of eating disorder suffer from anorexia nervosa • Average age of onset is 16–17 yrs • Highest mortality rate among psychiatric disorder in adolescence (medical complications and suicide) • 70% chance an identical twin will develop anorexia in their lifetime if one is diagnosed • In Western countries it affects 1% in women and 0.5% in men • 50% achieve full recovery with treatment • Higher rates of full recovery in adolescents and lower mortality compared to adults • 10:1 Female to male ratio

Table 17.2 Some common signs and symptoms of anorexia.

Psychological signs	Physical health symptoms	Physical/behavioural signs
Loss of appetite	Cardiovascular problems	Anaemia
Irritability	Weight loss	Tachycardia
Poor concentration	Amenorrhoea	Arrythmia
Poor memory	Impotence	Loss of sensation in extremities
Social withdrawal	Hypothalamic dysfunction	Some ritualistic behaviours
Insomnia	Osteoporosis	Dry and thin skin
Obsession	Thyroid dysfunction	Muscle atrophy
Depression	Lethargy	Breast atrophy
Anxiety	Dizziness/fainting	Dental problems (eroded enamel)
Low self-esteem	Hair loss	Brittle hair and nails
Low confidence	Cold extremities	
Loss of libido	Constipation	

Table 17.3 Diagnostic criteria.

1. Significantly low body weight of at least 15% below that expected for age height and build with 17.5 or less BMI. This may be through weight loss or never gaining weight.
2. Self-induced weight loss through avoidance (of fattening foods), excessive exercise, purging, vomiting, use of appetite suppressants, use of diuretics, and/or laxatives.
3. Cognitive distortion of body image in form of persistent and intrusive dread of fatness/weight gain with self-imposed low weight threshold.
4. Widespread endocrine disorder involving the hypothalamus, pituitary and/or adrenal glands. Effects on the gonadal axis manifests as amenorrhoea in women and, loss of sex drive and potency in men.
5. Delayed or arrested puberty if onset is prepubertal.

Long-term Conditions in Adults at a Glance, First Edition. Edited by Aby Mitchell, Barry Hill, and Ian Peate.
© 2023 John Wiley & Sons Ltd. Published 2023 by John Wiley & Sons Ltd.

Anorexia nervosa is a serious mental health condition within the eating disorder cluster. It is characterised by deliberate weight loss, self-induced and/or sustained by the patient (WHO 1992) through restrictive food intake and persistent extreme behaviours that interfere with weight gain associated with the intense fear of weight gain (NICE 2017). These behaviours are associated with psychological disturbances and include excessive preoccupation with body weight control. The typical onset of eating disorder is early-mid adolescence, but can emerge at any age. Statistical data can be seen in Table 17.1.

People with anorexia consistently restrict calory intake leading to significantly low body weight below the minimum for their age, sex, and health. Calorie intake is persistently not enough for the body's needs and leads to delayed or arrested growth in adolescence. A person with anorexia has distortions in perception of their own body. They deny severity of their behaviours and related risk. They may present with repetitive behaviours aimed at restricting calorie intake and/or compensatory behaviours aimed at ridding the body of ingested calories. Symptoms can be seen in Table 17.2.

Typical presentation include:

1 Behavioural – food restriction and ridding the body of ingested calories.

2 Psychological – body image disturbances/distorted perception and related distress prompting the compensatory behaviours and at times leading to other psychological co-morbidities.

3 Physical – weight loss and related medical complications.

Diagnostic criteria

Diagnosis is based on personal history corroborated by family/carer/friend, clinical evaluation and suggestive clinical features. It involves structured history taking, methodical detailed questioning with in-depth descriptions of personal accounts from the individual patient and those around them. This is complemented by clinical procedures and tests for an in-depth medical and evaluation of risk to aid effective treatment planning/interventions (see Table 17.3). Males are usually overlooked in diagnosis, hence the female–male ratio of 10:1. Instead male anorexic patients will be identified with such personality traits as persevering, obsessive-compulsive, self-critical, anxious or perfectionist.

Atypical anorexia

This is a diagnosis of anorexia where all symptoms included in the diagnosis are present except for weight which remains within normal range.

Support

Early assistance with a multi-professional and person-centred approach provides better treatment outcomes. Most treatments for anorexia involve biological/pharmacological, behavioural and psycho-social interventions delivered simultaneously and, as a result it is difficult to attribute success to a particular intervention (SIGN 2022). There is no evidence suggesting effective pharmacological treatments in children. Refeeding in anorexia in adults requires consideration of the starved physiology of the patient, their low body weight and abnormal electrolytes as these present high-risk factors if not adequately addressed. In severe and emergency situations, emergency room admission is considered if at risk of physical and/or psychological complications (NICE 2017). This is closely monitored due to risk related to electrolyte imbalance, e.g. hypophosphatemia. Pharmacological support includes refeeding. This is one of the medical interventions. Antidepressant medication is used to lift mood, treat anxiety, and stimulate appetite but medication should not be used as sole intervention.

Psychological treatment for anorexia nervosa in adults

It is important to consider one of the following after explaining what the treatments involve and helping them to choose their treatment of choice:

• Individual Eating-Disorder-focused Cognitive Behavioural Therapy (CBT ED) – typically consist of up to 40 sessions over 40 weeks, with twice-weekly sessions in the first two or three weeks.

• Maudsley Anorexia Nervosa Treatment for Adults (MANTRA) – typically consists of 20 sessions, with weekly sessions for the first 10 weeks, and a flexible schedule after this. Up to 10 extra sessions for people with complex problems.

• Specialist Supportive Clinical Management (SSCM) – typically consists of 20 or more weekly sessions (depending on severity).

If individual CBT-ED, MANTRA, or SSCM is unacceptable, contraindicated or ineffective for adults with anorexia nervosa, consider either: one of these three treatments that the person has not had before or eating-disorder-focused Focal Psychodynamic Therapy (FPT). FPT typically consists of up to 40 sessions over 40 weeks.

Psychological treatment for anorexia nervosa in children and young people

Consider anorexia-nervosa-focused family therapy for children and young people (FT-AN), delivered as single-family therapy or a combination of single and multi-family therapy. This gives the option of sessions separately from their family members or carers and together with their family members or carers.

Other eating disorders

Bulimia nervosa is characterised by episodes of overeating followed by extreme ways of, and excessive preoccupation with, the control of body weight. These result in extreme behaviours aimed at restricting the fattening effect of the ingested food. Binge/purge cycles in bulimia can dominate the sufferer's life. Binge eating disorder means that the sufferer eats excessively very large amounts of food over a very short period of time without feeling they are in control. This is not followed by any behaviours to get rid of the ingested food. Other specified feeding or eating disorders (OFSED) are eating disorders with symptoms that don't exactly fit into anorexia, bulimia or binge eating disorders.

Signs and symptoms

These are wide-ranged and manifest as psychological, physical ill-health, and can be observable on physical appearance. This may also include some ritualistic behaviours that maintain/worsen symptoms (see Table 17.2).

18 Arthritis

Emily Ashwell

Table 18.1 Patterns of arthritis presentation.

Mono arthritis	Oligo arthritis (≤5 joints involved)	Poly arthritis (≥5 joints involved)	
		Symmetrical	**Asymmetrical**
Septic arthritis	Crystal arthritis	Rheumatoid arthritis	Reactive arthritis
Crystal arthritis	Psoriatic arthritis	Osteoarthritis	Psoriatic arthritis
Osteoarthritis	Reactive arthritis	Viruses (hepatitis A, B, and C, mumps)	
Trauma (haem arthritis)	Ankylosing spondylitis		
	Osteoarthritis		

Table 18.2 A summary of other forms of arthritis and rheumatological conditions.

Condition	Brief overview
Psoriatic arthritis	A chronic inflammatory arthritis with psoriasis as the strongest risk factor.
Ankylosing spondylitis	A genetic chronic inflammatory arthritis predominantly affecting the sacroiliac joints and spine, and eventually leads to ankyloses due to calcification.
Reactive arthritis	An acute aseptic arthritis which often derived from gastrointestinal or genitourinary tract infections.
Gout	An inflammatory crystal arthritis caused by hyperuricaemia and the deposition of urate crystals in the synovial fluids of joints, bone and other tissues, frequently the hallux.
Calcium pyrophosphate disease	Another crystal arthritis, also known as pseudo gout, results from the deposition of calcium pyrophosphate crystals into the joint space.

Long-term Conditions in Adults at a Glance, First Edition. Edited by Aby Mitchell, Barry Hill, and Ian Peate.

Arthritis refers to the inflammation of a joint, which is frequently associated with pain and restricted movement. There are over 100 types of arthritis, two of the most common being osteoarthritis and rheumatoid arthritis which have been described in further detail below along with septic arthritis which causes the most rapid destruction of the joint. Over 10 million people in the UK are diagnosed with arthritis or other rheumatological conditions which also affect the joints (NHS 2018). Despite a high global prevalence, the exact aetiology of arthritis remains unclear therefore requiring further research.

Presentation of arthritis

The precise symptoms of arthritis experienced are dependent on diagnosis following investigations (such as blood tests) and will vary between individuals. Nevertheless, arthritis is often characterised by pain, stiffness, restricted movement, warmth, erythema, and inflammation in and around the affected joint. Generally inflammatory arthritic pain is worse after rest and subsides with activity, however mechanical pain (e.g. from osteoarthritis) is worsened by activity and improves following rest. See Table 18.1.

Management

There is no current cure for arthritis and treatment varies between types, however the general goals involve managing pain and quality of life. This is done by prescribing analgesia, medication which slows disease progression, physiotherapy, occupational therapy and surgical intervention. The earlier arthritis is diagnosed the earlier treatment can be implemented, which is associated with improved outcomes.

Osteoarthritis

Osteoarthritis is the clinical syndrome of joint pain alongside functional limitation, impairing quality of life (NICE 2020). Osteoarthritis has a clinically significant impact on 9.6% of men and 18% of women over the age of 60 years making it the most common form of arthritis worldwide. It is identifiable by damage to the cartilage and narrowed joint space, often in the hip, knee, hands, and spine. It results in painful and difficult movement followed by joint stiffness. This is caused by cartilage progressively roughening and thinning out, until subchondral bone is exposed which may then develop abnormal growth, osteophytes, and bone cysts. Osteoarthritis tends to develop from middle age but can occur at any age following an injury or alongside other rheumatological conditions. Other risk factors include being a woman and having a family history of osteoarthritis. In osteoarthritis initial management involves positive lifestyle changes, including local muscle strengthening exercise alongside general aerobic fitness, weight loss (if appropriate), and encouraging suitable footwear to be worn. Pain relief should also be prescribed beginning with paracetamol and/or topical analgesia before escalating according to the World Health Organization analgesic ladder. If pain and quality of life remains impaired surgery may be considered on an individual basis (NICE 2020).

Rheumatoid arthritis

Rheumatoid arthritis is an autoimmune chronic systemic inflammatory disorder, firstly affecting the synovial lining of the joints, before spreading to tendons and bursa. This results in painful swelling which alters the joints shape and may result in bone and cartilage breaking down as well as increasing the risk of tendon rupture. Rheumatoid arthritis tends to present symmetrically and affect multiple joints, for some it can also result in other tissues and organs problems, notably the heart, lungs, and eyes. In the UK, there are approximately 400 000 individuals with rheumatoid arthritis. Although it can affect people in any age group, often it develops in middle age with pre-menopausal women three times more likely to be affected than men. Other risk factors include family history, smoking, and diet. The target of rheumatoid arthritis treatment is to slow disease progression and reduce joint inflammation, subsequently minimising joint destruction using disease-modifying anti-rheumatic drugs (DMARDs). Individuals on DMARDs should be closely monitored for side-effects and therapy effectiveness, adjusting dosage as required. Steroids, hot or cold therapies and oral analgesia can also be used to control flare-ups of pain or stiffness (NICE 2018).

Septic arthritis

Septic arthritis is the acute infection of one or more joints, predominantly in the knee, hip, and shoulder. Septic arthritis often results from bacterial infection via direct inoculation (local cellulitis, osteomyelitis, and joint replacements) or haematogenous spread following other disease, such as urinary tract infections. Septic arthritis can cause joint destruction in under 24 hours and has a mortality rate of >11% therefore, should always be excluded in any acutely inflamed joint to enable prompt diagnosis and treatment. Septic arthritis has an estimated incidence of 2–10 cases per 100 000 of the UK population. Risk groups for septic arthritis include those who are immunocompromised, in the extremes of age, intravenous drug users, or have rheumatoid arthritis or other chronic diseases. Septic arthritis treatment involves antibiotics (tailored to the individual's synovial fluid joint analysis and blood cultures taken) intravenously for at least two weeks before switching to oral antibiotics for an additional four weeks, potentially alongside surgical debridement.

Arthritis in children

Although arthritis is frequently associated with older adults, it also affects children. In the UK alone, around 12 000 children have been diagnosed with arthritis. Childhood arthritis with unknown origins is known as juvenile idiopathic arthritis, although these patients can also be affected by other rheumatological conditions such as septic arthritis. Juvenile idiopathic arthritis is characterised by chronic pain and autoimmune inflammation in at least one joint for ≥6 weeks with onset prior to turning 16 years of age. It is more common is females especially those aged two to three years with a genetic predisposition.

A summary of other forms of arthritis is given in Table 18.2.

19 Asthma

Barry Hill

Figure 19.1 Pathophysiology of asthma. Source: Peate 2017, Figures 12.11 and 12.12, p. 339.

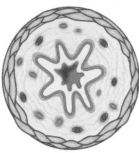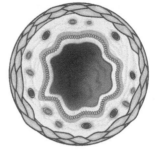

Asthma   Normal

Table 19.1 Patients at risk of developing near-fatal or fatal asthma.
Source: BTS and SIGN 2019.

A combination of severe asthma recognised by one or more of:
- previous near-fatal asthma, e.g. previous ventilation or respiratory acidosis
- previous admission for asthma, especially if in the last year
- requiring three or more classes of asthma medication
- heavy use of β2 agonist
- repeated attendances to A&E for asthma care, especially if in the last year.

AND adverse behavioural or psycho-social features recognised by one or more of:
- non-adherence with treatment or monitoring
- failure to attend appointments
- fewer GP contacts
- frequent home visits
- self-discharge from hospital
- psychosis, depression, other psychiatric illness, or deliberate self-harm
- current or recent major tranquilliser use
- denial
- alcohol or drug abuse
- obesity
- learning difficulties
- employment problems
- income problems
- social isolation
- childhood abuse
- severe domestic, marital, or legal stress

Asthma is a chronic respiratory condition associated with airway inflammation and hyper-responsiveness (NICE 2022). Asthma is a very common long-term condition that influences lung tissue and impacts on the normal mechanics of breathing. Asthma directly affects the airways that enable normal respiration and function of adequate oxygen into the lungs and carbon dioxide out of the lungs. In the UK, it is estimated that 5.4 million people have asthma (Asthma UK 2022). That's one in every 12 adults and one in every 11 children. People with asthma often have sensitive, inflamed airways. They can get symptoms like coughing, wheezing, feeling breathless or a tight chest. Asthma symptoms can come and go. Sometimes people may not have symptoms for weeks or months at a time. Asthma needs to be treated every day, even when feeling well, to lower the risk of symptoms and asthma attacks.

Pathophysiology

The pathophysiology of asthma is complicated and intricate. The bronchi and bronchioles contain smooth muscle and aligned with mucus secreting glands and ciliated cells (Figure 19.1). Once stimulated, mast cells release several cytokines which are chemical messengers that cause physiological changes to the lining of both bronchi and bronchioles. Cytokines are histamine, kinins, and prostaglandins, cause smooth muscle contraction increased mucus production and permeability. The airways narrow and become engorged with mucus and fluid from blood vessels causing narrowing of the airways (Figure 19.1) leading to increased work of breathing and respiratory effort for the patient.

Impact

Asthma is often under-diagnosed and under-treated, particularly in low- and middle-income countries. People with under-treated asthma can suffer sleep disturbance, tiredness during the day, and poor concentration. Asthma sufferers and their families may miss school and work, with financial impact on the family and wider community. If symptoms are severe, people with asthma may need to receive emergency health care and they may be admitted to hospital for treatment and monitoring. In the most severe cases, asthma can lead to death.

Causes

Many factors have been identified by the World Health Organization (WHO) (WHO 2022) which are specifically linked to an increased risk of developing asthma, although it is often difficult to find a single, direct cause. The pathophysiology of asthma can be seen in Figure 19.1. Asthma is more likely if other family members also have asthma – particularly a close relative, such as a parent or sibling.
• Asthma is more likely in people who have other allergic conditions, such as eczema and rhinitis (hay fever).
• Urbanisation is associated with increased asthma prevalence, probably due to multiple lifestyle factors.
• Events in early life affect the developing lungs and can increase the risk of asthma. These include low birth weight, prematurity, exposure to tobacco smoke and other sources of air pollution, as well as viral respiratory infections.
• Exposure to a range of environmental allergens and irritants are also thought to increase the risk of asthma, including indoor and outdoor air pollution, house dust mites, moulds, and occupational exposure to chemicals, fumes, or dust.

Children and adults who are overweight or obese are at a greater risk of asthma.

Signs and symptoms

Asthma is heterogeneous, with different underlying disease processes and variations in severity (Table 19.1), clinical course, and response to treatment. Asthma is characterised by symptoms including cough, wheeze, chest tightness, and shortness of breath, and variable expiratory airflow limitation, that can vary over time and in intensity. Symptoms can be triggered by factors including exercise, allergen or irritant exposure, changes in weather, and viral respiratory infections. Symptoms may resolve spontaneously or in response to medication and may sometimes be absent for weeks or months at a time (BTS and SIGN 2019). Exacerbations of asthma can occur and is a term used to describe the onset of severe asthma symptoms, which can be life-threatening.

Pharmacological management of asthma

Short-term management of asthma may prevent or relieve symptoms during acute episodes of wheeze and from asthma attack. They may be the only medicines needed for mild asthma or asthma that happens only with physical activity. These include:
• Inhaled short-acting beta2-agonists (SABAs) open the airways so air can flow through them during an asthma attack. Side-effects can include tremors and rapid heartbeat.
• Oral corticosteroids reduce swelling in the airways caused by severe asthma symptoms.
• Short-acting anticholinergics help open the airways quickly. This medicine may be less effective than SABAs, but it is an option for people who may have side effects from SABAs.

Corticosteroids (steroid hormone medicines) reduce inflammation in the body. They may be taken as a pill or inhaled. The pill form can have more serious side-effects than the inhaled form. Over time, high doses can raise the risk of cataracts (clouding of the eye) or osteoporosis. Osteoporosis makes bones weaker and more likely to break. Common side-effects from inhaled corticosteroids include a hoarse voice or a mouth infection called thrush. Biologic medicines may be prescribed for severe asthma. These include medicines such as benralizumab that are injected into a vein or below the skin.
• Leukotriene modifiers reduce swelling and keep airways open.
• Inhaled mast cell stabilisers, such as cromolyn, help prevent swelling in the airways when patients are around allergens or other asthma triggers.
• Inhaled long-acting bronchodilators, such as long-acting beta2-agonists (LABAs) or long-acting muscarinic antagonists (LAMAs), may be added to metre dose inhalers (MDIs) to prevent airways from narrowing.
• Allergy Injectables, called subcutaneous immunotherapy (SCIT), reduce the body's response to allergens.

20 Angina

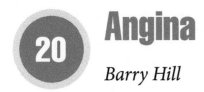

Barry Hill

Figure 20.1   Coronary artery disease showing healthy heart, angina pectoris, and myocardial infarction.

Coronary artery disease
angina pectoris and myocardial infarction

Healthy heart   **Angina pectoris**   **Myocardial infarction**

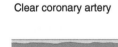

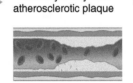

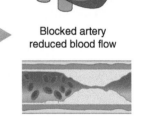

Myocyte damage

Clear coronary artery   Coronary artery with   Blocked artery
                           atherosclerotic plaque   reduced blood flow

A ngina is chest pain caused by reduced blood flow to the heart muscles; it is also called angina pectoris. Angina pain is often described as squeezing, pressure, heaviness, tightness, or pain in the chest. It may feel like a heavy weight lying on the chest. This is usually because of the arteries that supply the heart muscle have become hardened and narrowed. Most cases of angina are caused by atherosclerosis, which is a condition where the arteries become hardened and narrowed due to a build-up of fatty substances that are known as plaques. This can restrict the blood supply to the heart muscle and trigger the symptoms of angina. Conditions that affect the normal flow of blood, such as atherosclerosis, are known as cardiovascular diseases (CVD). Angina may be a new pain that needs to be checked by a health-care provider, or recurring pain that goes away with treatment. It is not usually life-threatening, but it is a warning sign of increased risk of a heart attack or stroke.

Types of angina

There are several types of angina including stable, unstable, vasospastic, and microvascular.

In stable angina, symptoms will usually develop gradually over time and follow a set pattern, for example, a person may only experience symptoms when climbing stairs or when they are under a lot of stress. Symptoms of stable angina usually only last for a few minutes and can be improved by resting and/or taking medication called glyceryl trinitrate (GTN). Stable angina is not considered to be life-threatening on its own, but is a sign that the arteries supplying blood to the heart muscle are narrowing. This means that there is an increased risk of experiencing more serious conditions, such as a heart attack.

In unstable angina, symptoms can develop rapidly and can persist even when a person is at rest. The symptoms may continue for some time. Symptoms of unstable angina might also not respond to treatment with GTN. People may experience symptoms of unstable angina after previously having symptoms of stable angina. However, unstable angina can also occur in people who have not had stable angina. Unstable angina should be regarded as a medical emergency because it is a sign that the blood supply to and the function of the heart is compromised, increasing the risk of having a heart attack. There are many different options for treatment for unstable angina, but it can often be treated with medication and/or types of surgical interventions.

Vasospastic angina, also known as coronary artery spasm or Prinzmetal's angina, is rare. It can happen during the night when resting, when a coronary artery supplying blood and oxygen to the heart goes into spasm and narrows or tightens and lets less blood through.

Microvascular angina (also known as cardiac syndrome X) usually happens when people are under physical pressure, for example when exercising, or when stressed or anxious. The pain is often caused by spasms in the smallest coronary arteries restricting blood flow.

Diagnosis and evaluation

To diagnose the cause of angina, the following tests may be performed:

Electrocardiogram (ECG): This test records the electrical activity of the heart, which is used to diagnose heart abnormalities such as arrhythmias or to show ischaemia (lack of oxygen and blood) to the heart.

Stress test without imaging: This heart-monitoring test is used to help evaluate how well the heart performs with activity. During a stress test, patients will usually be asked to perform physical exercise, such as walking on a treadmill. An ECG is recorded during the period of exercise. The ECG is assessed by the clinician to see if the heart reached an appropriate heart rate and if there were any changes to suggest decreased blood flow to the heart. If a patient is unable to perform exercise, medications that mimic the heart's response to exercise may be used.

Blood tests: The tests can identify certain enzymes such as troponin that leak into the blood after the heart has suffered severe angina or a heart attack. Blood tests can also identify elevated cholesterol, low-density lipoprotein (LDL) and triglycerides that place people at higher risk for coronary artery disease and consequently angina.

Treatments

Medication

The main medication used to prevent angina attacks is GTN which belongs to a group of medicines called nitrates that relax the muscle walls of the blood vessels and reduce the workload of the heart. GTN spray is used to treat angina at the onset of an attack. Additionally, there are two other types of medication that are used in the treatment of angina which include beta blockers – to make the heart beat slower and with less force, and calcium channel blockers to relax the arteries, increasing blood supply to the heart muscle. If a person cannot have either of these medicines, they may be given another medicine such as ivabradine, nicorandil, or ranolazine. Medicines to prevent hearts attacks and strokes may also be prescribed if the patient is at very high risk. These include a low dose of aspirin to prevent blood clots, statins to reduce cholesterol (blood fats) levels, and angiotensin converting enzymes (ACE inhibitors) to reduce blood pressure

Surgery

Surgery may be recommended if medicines are not helping control angina. The two main types of surgery for angina are coronary artery bypass graft (CABG) – a section of blood vessel is taken from another part of the body and used to reroute blood around a blocked or narrow section of artery; and a percutaneous coronary intervention (PCI, formerly known as angioplasty with stent). This is a non-surgical procedure that uses a catheter (a thin flexible tube) to place a small structure called a stent to open blood vessels in the heart that have been narrowed by plaque build-up, a condition known as atherosclerosis. Postoperatively patients are usually treated with low-dose aspirin clopidogrel, and an injection of a blood-thinning medicine. Additional surgery (either CABG or PCI) may be recommended if patients continue to have a high risk of having another angina attack, or high risk of having a heart attack or stroke.

Many people with angina have a good quality of life and continue as usual. Living an active lifestyle is also important to help prevent underlying coronary heart disease (Figure 20.1) from getting worse.

21 Anxiety

Louise Lingwood

Figure 21.1 Considerations for health and social-care professionals.

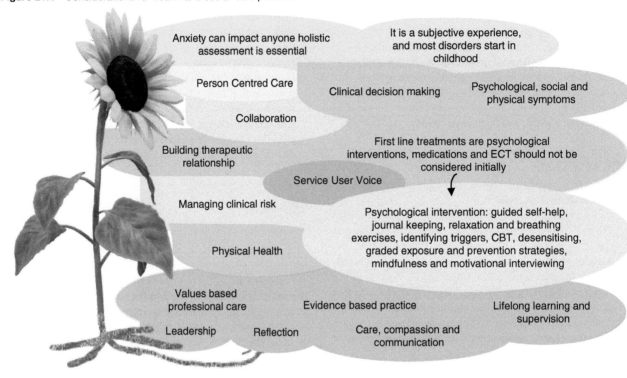

Anxiety can impact anyone holistic assessment is essential

It is a subjective experience, and most disorders start in childhood

Person Centred Care

Clinical decision making

Psychological, social and physical symptoms

Collaboration

Building therapeutic relationship

First line treatments are psychological interventions, medications and ECT should not be considered initially

Service User Voice

Managing clinical risk

Psychological intervention: guided self-help, journal keeping, relaxation and breathing exercises, identifying triggers, CBT, desensitising, graded exposure and prevention strategies, mindfulness and motivational interviewing

Physical Health

Values based professional care

Evidence based practice

Lifelong learning and supervision

Leadership

Reflection

Care, compassion and communication

Figure 21.2 Types of anxiety.

PTSD can result from indirect or direct exposure to a severe shock, accident or a traumatic event – leading to symptoms in four categories - intrusion, negative change to mood and thoughts, arousal and reactivity

GAD is characterised by relentless worry, unrealistic view of problems, tension, aches, fatigue, poor concentration, sleep and social functioning

Panic occurs with or without agoraphobia. Onset may be unexpected and sudden with no exposure to threat. Panic is often accompanied by physical symptoms – difficulty breathing, sweating and trembling.

OCD is characterised by patterns of unwanted thoughts and obsessions related to fears and over focus resulting in repetitive behaviours. **Obsessions** and **compulsions** often have themes – Can resemble Autistic Spectrum Disorder

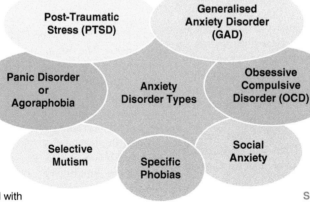

Post-Traumatic Stress (PTSD)

Generalised Anxiety Disorder (GAD)

Panic Disorder or Agoraphobia

Anxiety Disorder Types

Obsessive Compulsive Disorder (OCD)

Selective Mutism

Specific Phobias

Social Anxiety

Selective Mutism is associated with childhood anxiety disorder and evidence shows comorbidity for example with ADHD, OSD and social anxiety- shy, low self-esteem, exposure to trauma, may speak in comfortable social situations such as family home

Specific Phobias are characterised by intense irrational fear of a situation or object leading to avoidance or extreme distress

Social Anxiety is characterised by persistent fear of one or more social or performance situations. Fear of embarrassment, humiliation and/or being perceived negatively. It may lead to avoidance of social situations or situationally bound **panic attack**

What is anxiety?

It is normal to feel apprehensive, tense, or afraid at times. Anxiety is the body's natural response to managing stress or when facing potentially harmful events. In this sense, anxiety is protective, necessary for survival and motivates us to address problems, stay alert or take appropriate risks. When anxiety is difficult to control, intense or is pervasive and stops us doing things we enjoy it may be a sign that it is becoming a mental health issue or disorder. When left untreated anxiety disorder can become chronic in nature and associated with a negative course and outcome. Health and social-care professionals work across a variety of settings and will encounter people with an anxiety. All health and social-care professionals have a role to play in the prevention, assessment, diagnosis, and the management of anxiety (Figure 21.1).

Fight, fright, or freeze

When faced with an event that we perceive to be threatening or stressful it causes an automatic, physiological reaction, and the body prepares to 'fight, freeze, or run'. We have no control over this acute stress response. The bodies stress response involves both the nervous system and the endocrine system. The activity in our autonomic nervous system leads to several physiological changes within the body. These include increased respiration, pulse and blood pressure. In addition, the pupils dilate, and muscles tense. The processes of digestion and reproduction are suppressed, and we enter a fight, flight, or freeze state.

Anxiety disorder

Anxiety disorders are forms of emotional disorder and include generalized anxiety disorder (GAD), panic disorder, separation anxiety disorder, obsessive compulsive disorder (OCD), specific phobias, agoraphobia, and selective mutism (Figure 21.2). Anxiety can affect anyone at any age, but most disorders start in childhood, adolescence, or early adulthood.

Anxiety is a subjective experience that impacts psychological, social and physical health. It is essential to differentiate between an emotional disorder and a possible physical health condition as presentation of anxiety includes both psychological and physical symptoms. To meet the threshold diagnosis of an anxiety disorder, a certain number of symptoms must be experienced beyond a minimum specified period and cause considerable personal distress, with an associated impairment in day-to-day functioning. Anxiety symptoms often co-exist with other psychological symptoms, particularly depressive symptoms.

Clinical features

People with anxiety can experience a range of symptoms that are cognitive, behavioural and physical in nature dependent on the type of anxiety experienced (Figure 21.2). The predominant symptom of anxiety is excessive worry or fear. Symptoms can include:
* fear and avoidance
* feelings of doom or being in danger
* anger
* sleep disturbance
* irritability and restlessness
* inability to concentrate
* physical tension
* somatic symptoms – sweaty, numb or tingling hands or feet, nausea, abdominal discomfort, heart palpitations, and dizziness
* hyperventilation
* dry mouth (may be related to medication)
* hyperactivity
* hot flushes
* ruminating thoughts and compulsions.

Causes of anxiety

The development of anxiety disorder is complex and may include several factors such as environmental stressors, brain chemistry, genetic factors, chronic physical health conditions and substance misuse or withdrawal. The prevalence of anxiety in the general population is around 6% at any one time in the UK with GAD being the most common and OCD and panic disorder the least common. The coronavirus disease (COVID-19) pandemic is believed to have escalated the prevalence of anxiety as high as to 38% in the UK population.

Risk factors

The cause of anxiety is not yet clear, however there are several known risk factors which may increase a person's vulnerability:
* Family history: much debate as to whether this is an inherited tendency or if learnt responses arising from living with anxious people.
* Gender: women are twice as likely as men to be diagnosed with an anxiety disorder.
* Age: The average age of onset is 11 years of age.
  * More common in younger and middle-aged adults.
* Substance use or withdrawal: may heighten anxiety states.
* Life events: adverse childhood experiences or abuse, parental loss, employment issues or loss, domestic violence, excessive demands or high expectations.
* Chronic health issues.

Management

The stepped care approach consists of four evidence-based interventions which include watchful waiting, guided self-help, problem-solving treatment and referral to secondary care. Interventions are considered in collaboration with the individual and are dependent on the severity of symptoms and the diagnosis. Treatment guidance recommend evidence-based psychological interventions as the first line of treatment in preference to pharmacological intervention. Psychoeducation should be offered, and the presentation monitored, and the individual should be referred on for specialist assessment where necessary. Health Care Professional should consider signposting patients to social prescribing, pharmacological interventions, psychological wellbeing support strategies, and self help mechanisms.

Prevention

It is important to become aware of the triggers associated with the anxiety experienced so that it can be addressed. A balanced diet is essential for good health and well-being. Foods high in omega 3 fatty acids are known to reduce anxiety. Limiting caffeine intake is recommended and may irradicate or alleviate the symptoms experienced.

22 Atrial fibrillation

Barry Hill

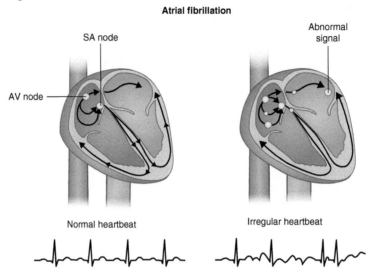

Figure 22.1 Atrial fibrillation.

Atrial fibrillation

SA node

AV node

Abnormal signal

Normal heartbeat

Irregular heartbeat

Table 22.1 The symptoms and impacts of AF[a].

- abnormal heart rhythm
- palpitations (feels like a racing, fluttering, flip flopping feeling in the chest)
- chest pain
- finding it harder to exercise
- tiredness
- shortness of breath
- dizziness or feeling faint
- sometimes people do not experience any symptoms and AF is detected when having a medical examination or check-up. This is common in older people.

Sometimes AF is:
- Occasional, lasting for minutes or hours. People may not need treatment if their heart rate returns to normal.
- Persistent and does not return to normal.
- Long-term persistent, which is continuous and lasts over a year.
- Permanent and does not go away. This indicates the need for regular medications or treatment to manage heart rate and prevent blood clots.

[a] Atrial flutter – Some people with atrial fibrillation also have atrial flutter. With atrial flutter the rhythm in the heart is less disorganised than with atrial fibrillation and it may feel milder. If this is the case, they may get periods of atrial flutter followed by periods of atrial fibrillation. People with atrial flutter are still at risk of further heart conditions or a stroke and may still need treatment.

Atrial fibrillation (AF) is a heart condition that causes an irregular and often abnormally fast heart rate (Figure 22.1). A normal heart rate should be regular and between 60 and 100 beats per minute when at rest. There are three different types of AF including paroxysmal, persistent, and permanent. Paroxysmal AF means that there are episodes of AF that come and go. Each episode comes on suddenly but will also stop suddenly without treatment within seven days (usually within two days). The heartbeat then goes back to a normal rate and rhythm. The period of time between each episode (each paroxysm) can vary greatly from case to case. Although paroxysmal AF means that it will stop on its own, some people with paroxysmal AF take treatment to stop it as quickly as possible after it starts. With persistent AF, it lasts longer than seven days and is unlikely to revert back to normal without treatment. However, the heartbeat can be reverted back to a normal rhythm with treatment. Persistent AF tends to come and go so it may come back again at some point after successful treatment. Finally, permanent AF is long-term, and the heartbeat does not return back to a normal rhythm. This may be because treatment has been tried and was not successful, or because treatment has not been tried. People with permanent AF are treated to bring their heart rate back down to normal but the rhythm remains irregular. The symptoms and impacts of AF can be seen in Table 22.1.

Aetiology

Atrial fibrillation (AF) is most associated with hypertension, coronary artery disease, and myocardial infarction. Other aetiologies include:

Cardiac or valve conditions, such as:
- Congestive heart failure
- Rheumatic valvular disease
- Atrial or ventricular dilation or hypertrophy
- Pre-excitation syndromes (such as Wolff–Parkinson–White syndrome)
- Sick sinus syndrome
- Congenital heart disease
- Inflammatory or infiltrative disease (such as pericarditis, amyloidosis, or myocarditis)

Non-cardiac conditions, such as:
- Acute infection
- Autonomic neuronal dysfunction (such as vagally induced AF)
- Electrolyte depletion (such as hypokalaemia and hyponatremia)
- Cancer (such as primary lung cancer involving the pleura and pericardium, and cancers such as breast cancer and malignant melanoma metastasising to the pericardium)
- Pulmonary embolism
- Thyrotoxicosis
- Diabetes mellitus

Dietary and lifestyle factors, such as:
- Excessive caffeine intake
- Alcohol abuse (especially in susceptible individuals such as those with structural heart disease)
- Obesity
- Smoking
- Medication exposure (such as thyroxine or bronchodilators)

Diagnosis

It is important to suspect atrial fibrillation (AF) in people with an irregular pulse, with or without any of the following symptoms, including breathlessness, palpitations, chest discomfort, syncope or dizziness, reduced exercise tolerance, malaise/listlessness, decrease in mentation, or polyuria. Also, it is important to recognise that a potential complication of AF includes stroke, transient ischaemic attack, and heart failure. Absence of an irregular pulse makes a diagnosis of AF unlikely, but its presence does not reliably indicate AF. Differential diagnoses of an irregular pulse include:
- Atrial flutter – characterised by a saw-tooth pattern of regular atrial activation on the electrocardiogram.
- Atrial extrasystoles – common and may cause an irregular pulse.
- Ventricular ectopic beats.
- Sinus tachycardia – sinus rhythm with more than 100 beats per minute.
- Supraventricular tachycardias, including atrial tachycardia, atrioventricular nodal re-entry tachycardia, and Wolff–Parkinson–White syndrome.
- Multifocal atrial tachycardia – often seen in people with severe pulmonary disease.
- Sinus rhythm with premature atrial or ventricular contractions.

Treatments

Anticoagulants

Anticoagulants stop blood from clotting and can help lower risk of having a stroke.

Direct-acting anticoagulants

Direct-acting anticoagulants such as rivaroxaban, dabigatran, apixaban, and edoxaban are recommended for people who have a high or moderate risk of having a stroke. Rivaroxaban, dabigatran, apixaban, and edoxaban do not interact with other medicines and do not require regular blood tests.

Warfarin

Warfarin is an anticoagulant that maybe offered if direct-acting anticoagulants are not suitable. There is an increased risk of bleeding in people who take warfarin, but this small risk is usually outweighed by the benefits of preventing a stroke. It is important to take warfarin as directed by the prescriber. People who take warfarin will need to have regular blood tests and dosage changes. Many medicines can interact with warfarin and cause serious problems. While taking warfarin, patients should be careful about drinking too much alcohol regularly and avoid binge drinking. Drinking cranberry juice and grapefruit juice can also interact with warfarin and is not recommended.

Cardioversion

Cardioversion may be recommended for some people with atrial fibrillation. It involves giving the heart a controlled electric shock to try to restore a normal rhythm. Cardioversion is usually carried out in hospital so the heart can be carefully monitored. When having had atrial fibrillation for more than two days, cardioversion can increase the risk of a clot forming. In this case, patients will be prescribed an anticoagulant for three to four weeks before cardioversion, and for at least four weeks afterwards to minimise the chance of having a stroke.

Catheter ablation

Catheter ablation is a procedure that very carefully destroys the diseased area of the heart and interrupts abnormal electrical circuits. It is an option if medicine has not been effective or tolerated. Catheters (thin, soft wires) are guided through one of the veins into the heart, where they record electrical activity. When the source of the abnormality is found, an energy source, such as high-frequency radio waves that generate heat, is transmitted through one of the catheters to destroy the tissue. The procedure can be quick, or it may take up to three or four hours and may be carried out under general anaesthetic. Although catheter ablation works for most people who have it, there is a small risk the procedure might not work, or symptoms might return after treatment. People may be given anti-arrhythmic medicines for three months after a catheter ablation to help stop symptoms coming back.

Pacemaker

A pacemaker is a small battery-operated device that is usually implanted in the chest, just below the collarbone. It is usually used to stop the heart beating too slowly, but in atrial fibrillation it may be used to help the heartbeat regularly. Having a pacemaker fitted is usually a minor surgical procedure carried out under a local anaesthetic. This treatment may be used when medicines are not effective or are unsuitable.

23 Bipolar affective disorder

Vishal Jugessur and Angela Childs

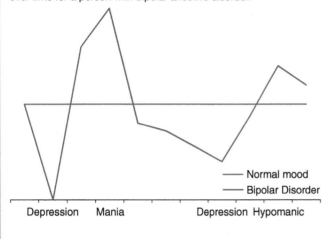

Figure 23.1 Visual representation of the different mood phases over time for a person with bipolar affective disorder.

- Normal mood
- Bipolar Disorder

Depression Mania Depression Hypomanic

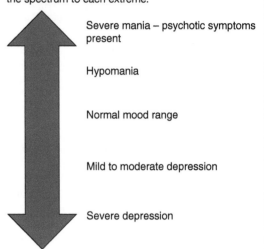

Figure 23.2 Severity of the phases of bipolar across the spectrum to each extreme.

Severe mania – psychotic symptoms present

Hypomania

Normal mood range

Mild to moderate depression

Severe depression

Definition

Bipolar affective disorder is described as a condition which affects your mood, making a person susceptible to having highs and lows, as well as possibly some psychotic symptoms during both these highs and lows. Bipolar disorder is associated with changes in activity or energy which can impact on the person's cognitive ability, their physical ability, and their behaviour.

Historically, the condition has been talked about for several years, as far back as the first century by Greek physicians. However, the two conditions were regarded as separate until the mid-nineteenth century when French psychiatrists created a separate new condition where the two extreme moods could be present at different times. The term 'manic depression' previously described this condition but in view of the stigma attached to anyone described as a 'maniac', in 1980, the Diagnostic and Statistical Manual III (DSM III) replaced the term manic depression with 'bipolar disorder'. There have been since further changes to the diagnosis, with bipolar type 1 and bipolar type 2 emerging.

Symptoms

Before looking at the two types of bipolar disorder, it is useful to consider the symptoms associated with the conditions.

Depression: Persistent extreme low mood, unable to find enjoyment, hopelessness, disturbed sleep, disturbed appetite, moving slower, or faster than usual, tiredness, feeling suicidal.

Mania: High energy levels, pressured speech, increased irritability, reckless behaviour, disinhibition, and possibly grandiose delusional beliefs, psychotic symptoms, decreased need for sleep, increased libido, with symptoms lasting seven days or more.

Hypomania: unlike mania, a hypomanic episode does not involve an evident loss of social functioning and does not have any psychotic symptoms. The symptoms must have been present for at least four days.

Figure 23.1 provides a visual representation of the different mood phases over time for someone with bipolar affective

Long-term Conditions in Adults at a Glance, First Edition. Edited by Aby Mitchell, Barry Hill, and Ian Peate.
© 2023 John Wiley & Sons Ltd. Published 2023 by John Wiley & Sons Ltd.

disorder. This figure is an example and the order and length of phases will differ for every individual. Figure 23.2 depicts the severity of the phases of bipolar across the spectrum to each extreme.

Variations

Bipolar disorder type 1 refers to a condition where the person has had at least one clear manic episode. The person may otherwise have episodes of depression, which are more likely than episodes of mania, in between periods of being well and fully recovered. A relapse into a manic phase of a bipolar disorder type 1 often involves significant risks and often requires hospitalisation.

Bipolar disorder type 2 refers to a condition where the person has had, in addition to the depressive episode(s), a hypomanic episode.

Prevalence and causes

The World Health Organization (WHO) states that in 2019, 40 million people in the world had experienced bipolar disorder. The average onset age is 25 years for bipolar disorder, and WHO report that bipolar disorder type 1 is more prevalent in men whilst bipolar type 2 is more prevalent in women.

A lot remains unknown of the cause of bipolar disorder, as in other mental health conditions, but that it appears the condition results from a combination of genetic factors and medical factors as well as external factors which include: environmental and social factors. Historical physical or sexual abuse in childhood can double the risk of developing bipolar disorder.

Treatment in a manic phase

As the condition is associated with instability of the mood, the conventional treatment option for bipolar affective disorder is from a class of medications known as mood stabilisers. The most established mood stabilisers are medicines like lithium, sodium valproate, carbamazepine, and lamotrigine. Often in pharmacology, particular medicines have several uses. Sodium valproate, carbamazepine, and lamotrigine are known as anti-convulsant drugs. In the same way, another treatment option for bipolar affective disorder is the use of anti-psychotic medications. Several of the anti-psychotic medications are licensed for use in the UK as mood stabilisers. The National Institute for Health and Care Excellence advises that if a person develops mania or hypomania and is not taking a mood stabiliser, then they should be offered an antipsychotic such as olanzapine, quetiapine, risperidone, or haloperidol. The anti-psychotics may show more rapid action in terms of managing acute symptoms of mania. If the patient was prescribed an anti-depressant, in a manic phase, this needs to be discontinued.

Risks in women of reproductive age

There have been warnings issued regarding the use of sodium valproate and its derivatives in women of reproductive age due to its association with severe birth defects, including spina bifida, face, and skull malformations and other developmental disorders

in babies from mothers who took the drug during pregnancy. Any clinicians who feel they have no alternative to prescribing sodium valproate to a woman of childbearing age must ensure that there is a pregnancy prevention programme in place and an annual review by a specialist and an annual risk assessment

Choice

The choice of medication should always involve the patient. Where this is not possible due to the patient's degree of illness, every effort should be made to include the patient in the discussions around treatment.

Prescriber's considerations

For the prescriber, it is vital to consider other existing conditions that the patient might suffer from, as well as medication sensitivity/allergies, medication interaction, and very importantly too, gender. The prescriber will need to discuss the therapeutic benefits, the side effects, and the known risks associated with specific treatments.

One important consideration a clinician in mental health often must take is regarding concordance to treatment. Where there is a high likelihood of somebody stopping their treatment, the consideration can be taken whether it may be better to prescribe an anti-psychotic in their long-acting depot injection form. Some patients prefer the option of having depot injections as this negates the need for them to be remembering to take tablets everyday of their lives.

Treatment in a depressive phase

Treatment of patients with a diagnosis of bipolar affective disorder who present as depressed need some careful consideration due to the risk of the person switching from depression into mania. This is commonly known a manic switch. There is little evidence that mood stabilisers help a person recover from a depressive phase, except for the antipsychotics such as olanzapine, quetiapine, and lurasidone. For this reason, an anti-depressant is often used when the person enters a depressive phase. Research indicates that patients with a diagnosis of bipolar affective disorder in a depressive phase are at high risk of switching from depression into mania in the group solely being treated on an anti-depressant medication compared to no risk of this switch in the group being treated on both an anti-depressant and a mood-stabiliser.

The challenges that present in treating bipolar disorder

In an acute manic phase, the patient often presents with poor insight and can present with challenging disinhibited and violent behaviour which often results in detention under the mental health act and hospitalisation. On the contrary, someone in a hypomanic phase may not come to the attention of services and go undetected, however, the associated behaviours may result in difficulties in various aspects of life.

There is a high prevalence of addiction in bipolar disorder and substance misuse can affect risk as well as clinical outcomes.

Bulimia nervosa

24

Tichaona Mubaira and Lucy Saunders

Other Eating Disorders

- Anorexia nervosa – Deliberate and sustained weight loss maintained through restrictive food intake and persistent extreme behaviours that interfere with weight gain and associated with intense fear of gaining weight with a BMI of typically below 17.5.
- Binge eating disorder – the sufferer eats excessively a very large amount of food over a very short period of time without feeling they are in control. This is not followed by any behaviours to get rid of the ingested food.
- Other specified feeding or eating disorder (OFSED) – eating disorder with symptoms that do not exactly fit into anorexia, bulimia, or binge eating disorders.

Table 24.1 Disorder and bulimia nervosa.

Eating disorders in general	Bulimia nervosa specifically
• 1.25–3.4 million people affected in the UK • 25% of those affected are male • Most commonly develop during adolescence • Most common in 16–40 yrs old • More likely to develop if there is family history • Highest mortality rates among psychiatric disorders • Better chances of recovery if appropriate treatment initiated earlier • Equal distribution across social classes	• Around 40% of people affected by eating disorder experience bulimia nervosa • Average age of onset is 18–19 yrs • Longer term effects of bulimia can be extremely damaging both physically and mentally • Early interventions and treatment can be very effective

Table 24.2 Some of the common signs and symptoms of bulimia.

Psychological signs	Physical health symptoms	Physical/behavioural signs
Preoccupation with eating Irresistible food cravings Morbid fear of fatness Social withdrawal Obsession Depression Anxiety Low self-esteem Low confidence	Cardiovascular problems Constipation Electrolyte disturbance Cardiac failure (with sudden death) Arrythmias Oesophageal erosion from excessive vomiting Pancreatitis Gastric ulcers Dental erosion Cold extremities Haematemesis Lethargy/fatigue	Bingeing on food Bloating Acid wear on knuckles Some ritualistic behaviours (compensatory behaviours) Dry and thin skin Dental problems (eroded enamel)/teeth sensitivity Healthy weight may be maintained Substance use problems especially in men Mouth ulcers

Overview (prevalence, description of the disorder)

Bulimia nervosa is an eating disorder cluster characterised by periods of overeating and behaviours to mitigate the fattening effect of the ingested food. An individual with bulimia nervosa would typically engage in binge eating, after which they may become preoccupied by the effects of the ingested food on the body/weight and would adopt extreme compensatory behaviours. Unlike anorexia nervosa, the body weight of an individual with bulimia may fall within the normal range of their age and build.

Typical features in bulimia nervosa:

1 Binge eating – sense of loss of control in their behaviour. Repeated episodes of eating more food in a single episode than would people of the same age, build, and in their circumstance would eat.

2 Compensatory behaviours – mainly purging by vomiting but also may include or alternatively use laxatives, diuretics, periods of fasting, extreme dieting, and/or extreme exercise.

3 Psychological – preoccupied by body image especially weight and shape prompting the compensatory behaviours and at times leading to other psychological co-morbidities.

4 Physical – not necessarily underweight as can maintain healthy weight for age and build. Potential acid wear on finger knuckles from inducing purging, and dentition examination may reveal enamel erosion from gastric acid.

Prevalence/statistical information

Table 24.1 provides an overview of the prevalence of eating disorders and bulimia.

Signs and symptoms

These are wide-ranged and manifest as psychological, physical ill-health and can be observed during physical examination. This may also include some ritualistic behaviours that maintain/worsen symptoms. Table 24.2 outlines some of the common signs and symptoms of bulimia. Some of the symptoms described may be similar to anorexia but of less severity.

Diagnostic criteria

Diagnosis is based on personal history corroborated by family/carer/friend, clinical evaluation, and suggestive clinical observations. It involves structured history taking, methodical detailed questioning with in-depth descriptions of personal accounts from the individual patient and those around them. Bulimia may be a sequel to anorexia. This is complemented by clinical procedures and investigations for an in-depth medical assessment and evaluation of risk to aid effective treatment planning/interventions. For a definite diagnosis, all of the following are required:

1 Episodes of binge-eating resulting from persistent preoccupation with eating and irresistible food craving.

2 Attempts to counter fattening effects of ingested food by inappropriate compensatory behaviours such as self-induced vomiting and/or purgative abuse, follow on food restriction, drug use (laxatives, diuretics, appetite suppressants, thyroid preparations).

3 Morbid dread of fatness with a self-imposed low body weight threshold well below premorbid weight.

Atypical bulimia nervosa

This is a diagnosis of bulimia in which one or more key features is absent, but the individual presents a fairly typical clinical picture, e.g. an individual with normal or overweight but presenting with typical episodic overeating followed by self-induced vomiting or purging.

Lived experience perspective

> The more I denied my body the food it needed, the deeper my hunger became, and the greater the sense of control I felt being restored. One day the hunger finally overwhelmed me. I began to purge. This quickly developed into a dangerous cycle of binge eating and vomiting.
>
> *Person living with bulimia*

Recovery/interventions/treatment

In eating disorders early help with a person-centred approach provides better treatment outcomes. Bulimia nervosa-focused guided self-help provides self-control and better outcomes. Selective serotonin reuptake inhibitor anti-depressants are used in treating resultant depression-related symptoms although there is no evidence suggesting effective pharmacological treatments especially in children. There is no evidence that hospitalisation has better outcomes either apart from the management, especially of acute suicidality.

Psychological treatment for bulimia nervosa in adults

Psychological treatments have a limited effect on body weight for people with bulimia nervosa.

Consider bulimia-nervosa-focused guided self-help for adults with bulimia nervosa. Such programmes should use cognitive behavioural self-help materials for eating disorders. Supplement the self-help programme with brief supportive sessions of 4–9 sessions lasting 20 minutes each over 16 weeks, running weekly at first.

If guided self-help is ineffective after four weeks, unacceptable or contraindicated, consider individual eating-disorder-focused cognitive behavioural therapy. This typically consists of up to 20 sessions over 20 weeks, with consideration for twice-weekly sessions in the first phase.

Psychological treatment for bulimia nervosa in children and young people

Consider bulimia-nervosa-focused family therapy for children and young people (FT-BN) of 18–20 sessions delivered over six months. Using psychoeducation with non-blaming approaches aimed at minimising compensatory behaviours. Individual eating disorder-focused cognitive behavioural therapy is also recommended where FT is contraindicated.

25 Bronchiectasis

Barry Hill

Table 25.1 Forms of bronchiectasis.

1. Cylindrical bronchiectasis is the mildest form and reflects the loss of the normal tapering of the airways. The symptoms may be quite mild, like a chronic cough, and usually are discovered on CT scans of the chest.
2. Saccular bronchiectasis is more severe, with further distortion of the airway wall and symptomatically, affected persons produce more sputum.
3. Cystic bronchiectasis is the most severe form of bronchiectasis, and fortunately it is the least common form. This often occurred in the pre-antibiotic era when an infection would run its course and the patient would survive with residual lung damage. These patients often would have a chronic productive cough, bringing up a cup or more of discoloured mucus each day. Bronchiectasis also may be congenital or acquired.

Figure 25.1 Representation of the cycle that leads to development of bronchiectasis. Source: Maselli et al. (2017).

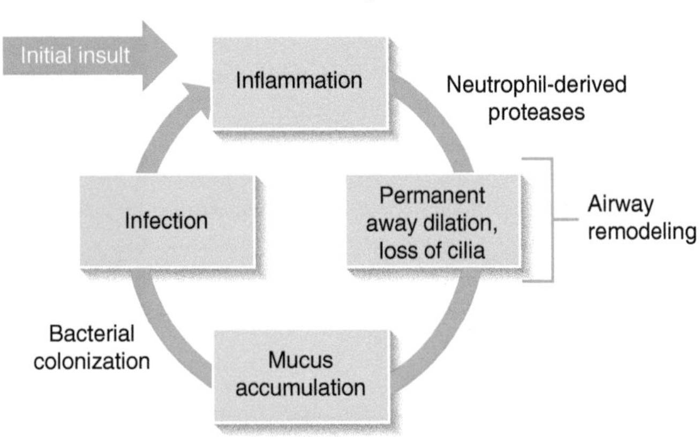
Bronchiectasis Cycle
Initial insult
Inflammation
Neutrophil-derived proteases
Permanent away dilation, loss of cilia
Airway remodeling
Mucus accumulation
Bacterial colonization
Infection

Table 25.2 Suspect bronchiectasis in adults (NICE 2022).

- Persistent production of mucopurulent or purulent sputum, particularly with relevant associated risk factors for bronchiectasis.
- A cough that persists for longer than 8 wk, especially with sputum production or a history of an appropriate trigger (over 90% of people).
- Rheumatoid arthritis if they have symptoms of chronic productive cough or recurrent chest infections.
- COPD with frequent exacerbations (two or more annually) and/or a positive sputum culture for *Pseudomonas aeruginosa* (or another potentially pathogenic organism) whilst stable.
- Asthma that is severe or poorly controlled.
- Inflammatory bowel disease and chronic productive cough.

Long-term Conditions in Adults at a Glance, First Edition. Edited by Aby Mitchell, Barry Hill, and Ian Peate.

Formerly regarded as a rare disease, bronchiectasis is now increasingly recognised and a renewed interest in the condition is stimulating drug development and clinical research. Bronchiectasis represents the final common pathway of several infectious, genetic, autoimmune, developmental, and allergic disorders and is highly heterogeneous in its aetiology, impact, and prognosis. Bronchiectasis is chronic airway dilation caused by chronic inflammation. The inflammation is often caused by inadequate clearance of microorganisms or chronic/frequent lung infections. Patients with bronchiectasis have thickened bronchial walls and suffer frequent sputum production and chronic coughs. It's important to recognise that bronchiectasis is uncommon. It is estimated around 1 in every 100 adults in the UK have the condition. It can affect anyone at any age, but symptoms do not usually develop until middle age. There are three primary types of bronchiectasis. These types are described by their anatomical appearance (Table 25.1).

Pathophysiology

In bronchiectasis, lung function deteriorates over many years. Patients become locked in a vicious cycle of infection, inflammation, and damage. Once infected the patient's inability to clear the pathogen leads to an inflammatory response. While inflammation protects against pathogens, in patients unable to clear microorganisms the inflammatory response may become chronic and counter-productive, leading to bronchial wall damage and irreversible dilatation of the airways (see Figure 25.1).

Signs and symptoms

Some of the most common symptoms are:
- Persistent cough
- Coughing with mucous production
- Coughing up mucus that has blood in it (known as haemoptysis)
- Chest pain or tightness
- Wheezing
- Clubbing of nails
- Loss of weight
  Flare-ups that usually include:
- Fatigue
- Fevers and/or chills
- Increased shortness of breath
- Night sweats

Risk factors/causes

The most common causes of bronchiectasis are cystic fibrosis and childhood respiratory disease. Other risk factors include viral, bacterial, and fungal infections, aspiration, airway obstruction, inhalation of toxic substances and immunosuppression. Many lung conditions, such as chronic obstructive pulmonary disease (COPD), allergic bronchopulmonary aspergillosis and bronchiolitis, can lead to the development of bronchiectasis, as can autoimmune or inflammatory disorders such as coeliac disease, rheumatoid arthritis, systemic lupus erythematosus, ankylosing spondylitis, Sjögren's syndrome and inflammatory bowel disease. Patients with congenital conditions may also be at risk, especially cardiorespiratory disease such as Marfan's syndrome, tracheobronchomegaly, pulmonary ciliary dyskinesia or chest wall deformities such as scoliosis and pectus excavatum.

There are several advisory symptoms that should arouse suspicion of bronchiectasis in adult patients (Table 25.2).

Recommendations for practice

If bronchiectasis is suspected:
- Take a thorough history.
  Arrange the following investigations:
1 Sputum culture – to identify colonising pathogens. Public Health England gives detailed guidance on the collection and transport of respiratory tract specimens.
2 Chest X-ray – to exclude other pathology and to help confirm the diagnosis where disease is severe.
3 Spirometry – to assess the severity of airflow obstruction and identify any co-existent diagnoses (such as COPD).
4 Oxygen saturation levels.
5 Full blood count including differential white cell count.
6 Other investigations – guided by clinical findings to confirm or rule out underlying causes for bronchiectasis.
- Assess for the presence of anxiety or depression, particularly in people who have severe breathlessness.
- Document the person's smoking history – if they currently smoke, offer support to stop.
- Measure the person's weight and calculate and document the person's body mass index (weight in kg/height in m²).
- Refer all people with suspected bronchiectasis to a respiratory consultant for investigations to confirm the diagnosis and determine the underlying cause, and for appropriate treatment.

Treatment

Bronchiectasis is often treated with medication, and patients may require respiratory physiotherapy. It suggested that patients stay well-hydrated: fluid supports the prevention of mucus thickening, which prevents sufficient ability to expectorate any mucous.

Medications may include:
- Antibiotics to treat any infection.
- Bronchodilators to relax the airway muscles and make breathing easier.
- Inhaled steroids to decrease any inflammation (often combined in the same inhaler as bronchodilators).
- Expectorants and mucus thinners to loosen the mucus in the lungs and make it easier to expectorate.
- Decongestants to ease congestion.

Chest physiotherapy is another important part of treatment. It includes percussion of the chest wall to loosen the mucus from the lungs. Patients may also be taught special breathing methods. These can move the mucus into the upper part of the airway so that it can be expectorated. Some patients may require oxygen therapy due to prolonged hypoxia and associated symptoms. In rare cases, surgical intervention is required including lung transplant. A patient's treatment plan will depend on the severity of their symptoms and other health conditions. Early diagnosis and treatment can stop the condition from getting worse. Some congenital causes of bronchiectasis include cystic fibrosis, Kartagener syndrome, Young's syndrome and alpha-1-antitrypsin deficiency. There are also acquired causes of bronchiectasis, which include: recurrent infection, aspiration of foreign bodies or other materials, inhaling toxic gases like ammonia, alcohol and drug abuse, tuberculosis, and inflammatory bowel disease (ulcerative colitis, Crohn's disease).

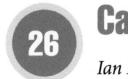

26 Cancer

Ian Peate

Figure 26.1 People with cancer in the UK. Source: Macmillan Cancer Support (2015a,b).

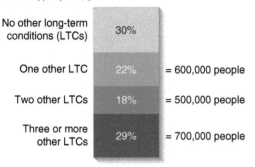

No other long-term conditions (LTCs)	30%	
One other LTC	22%	= 600,000 people
Two other LTCs	18%	= 500,000 people
Three or more other LTCs	29%	= 700,000 people

Figure 26.2 Cancer and co-existing conditions. Source: McConell et al. (2015).

Hypertension 42%
Obesity 31%
Mental health issues 21%
People living with cancer in the UK in mid-2014
Chronic Heart Disease 19%
Diabetes 14%
Arthritis 16%
Chronic Kidney Disease 17%

Figure 26.3 Three broad cancer groups. Source: McConnell et al. (2015).

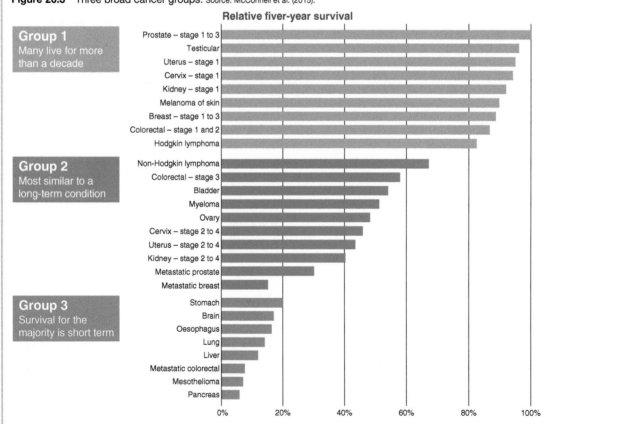

Relative fiver-year survival

Group 1 Many live for more than a decade
- Prostate – stage 1 to 3
- Testicular
- Uterus – stage 1
- Cervix – stage 1
- Kidney – stage 1
- Melanoma of skin
- Breast – stage 1 to 3
- Colorectal – stage 1 and 2
- Hodgkin lymphoma

Group 2 Most similar to a long-term condition
- Non-Hodgkin lymphoma
- Colorectal – stage 3
- Bladder
- Myeloma
- Ovary
- Cervix – stage 2 to 4
- Uterus – stage 2 to 4
- Kidney – stage 2 to 4
- Metastatic prostate
- Metastatic breast

Group 3 Survival for the majority is short term
- Stomach
- Brain
- Oesophagus
- Lung
- Liver
- Metastatic colorectal
- Mesothelioma
- Pancreas

0%   20%   40%   60%   80%   100%

Long-term Conditions in Adults at a Glance, First Edition. Edited by Aby Mitchell, Barry Hill, and Ian Peate.
© 2023 John Wiley & Sons Ltd. Published 2023 by John Wiley & Sons Ltd.

Cancer and long-term conditions

Multi-morbidity (long-term conditions) are known to contribute to the complexity of care for those people with cancer. There are more than 200 different types of cancer. Those with cancer experience multi-modal treatments, that is, treatments for multiple long-term conditions, as well as challenges related to navigating the health-care system.

There are significant challenges that people with long-term conditions and cancer have to face in terms of being able to strike a fine balance between their acute health needs and any underlying long-term conditions. These people can often experience unforeseen treatment complications, they have to negotiate silos across medical specialties and have to navigate and engage with those in the social care sector.

Patients should expect a more personalised care approach and to be included in multidisciplinary team meetings (see Chapter 9). There is an impetus to offer more effective integrated care across diseases; this will enhance person-centred care, patient experience, patient outcomes and provide support to those who are struggling to balance competing needs when they face multi-morbidity.

The number of adults diagnosed with cancer who concurrently have one or more chronic conditions is growing. Ageing is correlated with a higher incidence of cancer and other age-related chronic conditions, for example, diabetes, chronic obstructive pulmonary disease, heart disease, arthritis, and hypertension.

Incidence

Living with other long-term conditions as well as cancer reduces an individual's chance of survival and also increases the level of support they need. It is estimated that there are around 3 million people in the UK living with cancer. This number is expected to increase to 4 million in by 2030 and to 5.3 million by 2040. This increase can be attributed to the UK's growing and ageing population as well as improvements in cancer diagnosis and treatments.

In 2015 it was estimated that 1.8 million people were living with one or more other potentially serious long-term health conditions in addition to cancer – more than two in three (70%) of those with cancer.

The burden of long-term health conditions

The burden associated with a cancer diagnosis is often significant, with medical care becoming increasingly complex, usually involving a number of health-care specialties. These challenges are amplified when patients also have to cope with additional chronic health conditions.

Nearly 75% of people with cancer in the UK are also living with one or more other potentially serious long-term health condition. Around half have two or more conditions as well as cancer and more than one in four (29%) have three or more conditions as well as cancer (see Figure 26.1).

The top five most common long-term conditions for people with cancer are (see Figure 26.2):
1 Hypertension
2 Obesity
3 Mental health problems
4 Chronic heart disease
5 Chronic kidney disease.

The top four conditions noted are also the most common long-term conditions that affect those people without cancer. People with cancer however, are more likely than those without cancer to be living with one or more other long-term conditions; on average those with cancer are older than those who have never had cancer.

People with cancer are more likely than people without cancer to have hypertension. It has been suggested that hypertension can be linked with an increased risk of developing specific types of cancer, this may be due to lifestyle factors, for example, poor diet and a lack of exercise, increasing the risk of both conditions. There are some cancer treatments that may also increase the risk of hypertension. Those with cancer are also more likely to have chronic kidney disease than people without cancer. This may be due to shared risk factors or the long-term effects of some cancer treatments.

Those women with breast cancer and men with prostate cancer who have only one other serious long-term health condition prior to a diagnosis of cancer are more likely to die within seven years of diagnosis than those who do not have a pre-existing condition.

Three cancer groups

Figure 26.3 describes the three groups using survival rates for different cancers. The longer-term survival group includes cancers where 90% or more people live one year or more after a cancer diagnosis. More than 80% go on to live five years or more and many go on to live at least a decade. The shorter-term survival group includes cancers where fewer than 50% of people survive a year. The intermediate group experience moderate survival (one-year survival is over 50% but less than 90%).

The cancer group a patient is in will have an effect on their care trajectory. For those in the intermediate group this may mean that they face an exceptionally uncertain future with their ongoing complex care needs. This group may need a balance of acute intervention, self management and chronic illness management

People with cancer in the longer-term survival group may have fewer hospital admissions that are directly related to their cancer, many however will still be living with the consequences of cancer and its treatment. There will be some who will still face recurrence or second primary cancer years after primary treatment. Self-management with appropriate support is important, as well as a focus on impact of recovery and late effects and reducing unnecessary over-treatment.

Early diagnosis and effective treatment or palliative care is important in supporting those people with shorter-term survival cancer.

The care required for people living with cancer and long-term conditions extends beyond acute care. Understanding the full extent of the needs of those living with cancer and how care can be coordinated to best meet these needs is essential. Each person with cancer is different and the support that they require has to be tailored to their individual needs. Insight regarding the three groups identified in Figure 26.3 can help explain the complexity, intensity and longevity of needs for people with different cancer types and long-term conditions. Meeting the patients' informational, psychosocial, physical and coordination needs is paramount.

27 Chronic fatigue syndrome

Roberta Borg

Table 27.1 Aetiology and risk factors for CFS.

Genetics	Family history and twin registry studies show an increased familial/genetic predisposition.
Infection	50–80% of patients describe flu-like symptoms/viral illness prior to disease. Epstein–Barr virus, human herpes virus and human parvovirus all hypothesised to trigger the disease. COVID-19 – several studies observed similar symptoms to ME/CFS in patients with long-COVID syndrome.
Altered immune system	Observation studies show altered B cell subset levels, elevated levels of immunoglobulin G and autoantibodies in patients with ME/CFS.
Stress	Physical (physiological injury/surgery) and severe emotional/psychological stress.

Table 27.3 Investigations of a patient with suspected ME/CFS.

History	Identify presenting complaints, symptoms and onset. Past medical history, surgical history, drug history, co-morbidities, recent illness/surgery/stressful event.
Physical examination	Rigorous physical examination to assess for and pick up symptoms.
Psychosocial assessment	An assessment of the impact of symptoms on psychological and social well-being.
Investigations to exclude other diagnoses (a non-exhaustive list)	Urinalysis for protein, blood and glucose. Full blood count Urea and electrolytes Liver function Thyroid function Erythrocyte sedimentation rate or plasma viscosity C-reactive protein Calcium and phosphate Hb1Ac Serum ferritin Coeliac screening Creatine kinase vitamin D, vitamin B_{12} and folate levels Serological tests if there is a history of infection; and 9 a.m. cortisol for adrenal insufficiency.

Table 27.2 Symptoms experienced by ME/CFS patients.

Symptom	Description
Fatigue[a]	*Debilitating* fatigue worsened by activity, not caused by excessive exertion and not significantly relieved by rest.
Post-exertional malaise[a]	A decline after activity. Often delayed in onset by hours or days, is disproportionate to the activity, has a prolonged recovery time that may last hours, days, weeks or longer.
Unrefreshing sleep/sleep disturbance[a]	Broken or shallow sleep, altered sleep pattern or hypersomnia. Patients feeling exhausted, achy, and stiff on waking.
Cognitive difficulties[a]	Sometimes described as 'brain fog'. May include problems finding words, difficulty speaking, slowed responsiveness, short-term memory problems and difficulty concentrating or multi-tasking.
Pain	There is a significant degree of myalgia. Pain can be experienced in the muscles and/or joints and is often widespread and migratory in nature. Often patients complain of headaches (of new type, pattern, or severity), eye pain, abdominal pain.
Autonomic manifestations	Orthostatic intolerance – neurally mediated hypotension (NMH), postural orthostatic tachycardia syndrome (POTS), postural hypotension; light-headedness, nausea and irritable bowel syndrome; urinary frequency and bladder dysfunction; palpitations, exertional dyspnoea.
Neuroendocrine manifestations	Loss of thermostatic stability resulting in profuse sweating, chills, hot flushes or feeling very cold. Intolerance of extremes of heat or cold.
Immune manifestations	Tender lymph nodes, recurrent sore throat, recurrent flu-like symptoms, general malaise, new sensitivities to food, medications and/or chemicals.

[a] Predominant symptoms.

Figure 27.1 The proposed aetiology, pathophysiological pathways and associated symptoms – original diagram by Roberta Borg.

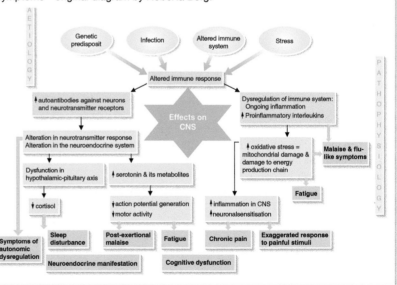

Long-term Conditions in Adults at a Glance, First Edition. Edited by Aby Mitchell, Barry Hill, and Ian Peate.
© 2023 John Wiley & Sons Ltd. Published 2023 by John Wiley & Sons Ltd.

Chronic fatigue syndrome, also known as myalgic encephalomyelitis and often referred to as ME/CFS, is a complex, long-term condition that is thought to affect over 250 000 people in England and Wales. Its aetiology remains poorly understood and its diagnosis a challenge.

ME/CFS affects multiple body systems and is often characterised by severe fatigue, cognitive difficulties, sleep disturbance, autonomic dysfunction, and post-exertional malaise. It affects everyone differently and its impact varies widely. Severity is often described as mild/moderate/severe/very severe, depending on the level of impact of symptoms on everyday functions. For some people, symptoms still allow them to carry out daily activities, whereas for others they are profoundly disabling.

There is no cure for ME/CFS and the treatment focuses on management of symptoms as well as managing the patients' and carers' expectations. This can be particularly challenging because of the fluctuating nature of the condition, where symptoms can change unpredictably.

Epidemiology

The *estimated* prevalence is 0.1–0.5%. The disease predominantly affects adults with a peak age of onset between 20 and 45 years and a female to male ratio of 3 : 1. It affects all racial/ethnic groups and is seen across all socioeconomic strata although it seems to have a higher incidence in socially deprived families.

Aetiology and risk factors

The aetiology of ME/CFS is complex and remains poorly understood. There are several theories supporting an interplay of genetics, infection and altered immunology as well as stressful events in relation to the causation of ME/CFS (see Table 27.1).

Pathophysiology and symptoms

The pathophysiology of ME/CFS is still being investigated. Figure 27.1 illustrates some of the proposed pathophysiological pathways and their associated symptoms, while Table 27.2 gives a more detailed description of the symptoms experienced by these patients.

Diagnosis

There is no diagnostic test for ME/CFS; it is established on clinical grounds alone, by recognising a set of symptoms. Following a rigorous review of the evidence and analysis of the existing diagnostic criteria in the literature, the NICE guidelines propose that:
1 ME/CFS should be diagnosed in a child, young person or adult who has the predominant four symptoms (marked by [a] in Table 27.2), which have persisted for three months and are not explained by another condition.
2 Health-care professionals should seek advice from an appropriate specialist to confirm diagnosis and develop a care and support plan.

3 Children and young people should be referred directly to a paediatric ME/CFS specialist to confirm their diagnosis and develop a care and support plan.

Typically, investigations of a patient with suspected ME/CFS begin with a history and physical examination, focusing on identifying the underlying symptoms and ruling out any other illnesses (Table 27.3).

Communication throughout the diagnostic process

Explain to people with suspected ME/CFS that their diagnosis can only be confirmed after three months of persistent symptoms. Reassure them that they can return for a review before that if they develop new or worsened symptoms and ensure that they know who to contact for advice. Provide information to people with ME/CFS and their family/carers. Recognise that patients may have experienced prejudice and may feel stigmatised by others who do not understand their illness.

Management/treatments

There is no cure for chronic fatigue syndrome. Treatment focuses on symptom management and relief, and care-plans are largely dependent on the severity of symptoms. The following are a few treatment strategies that may be included in individual care-plans:

Energy management – a self-management strategy where patients learn how to best utilise their energy levels in their daily lives. The treatment plan is put together with health-care professionals from an ME/CFS specialist team. It should include all types of activity (physical, cognitive, emotional, and social). An exercise plan may be suitable for some; graded exercise therapy (GET) is no longer recommended for everyone with ME/CFS.

Medical treatment – specific medicines may be prescribed to manage certain symptoms like pain, sleep disturbance, depression/anxiety and orthostatic intolerance.

Cognitive behaviour therapy – can help individuals change the way they think and behave and may help to reduce the distress associated with having a chronic illness.

Manage flare-ups/relapse – identify possible cause or triggers such as acute illness or overexertion. May need to reassess care-plan and temporarily reduce activity levels and increase frequency or duration of rest periods. Medically manage new symptoms if required/appropriate.

Prognosis

The outcome is very variable and often dependent on the severity of symptoms at the time of onset. Whilst some people improve over time, especially with treatment, others do not make a full recovery and will need to adapt to living with ME/CFS. Children and adolescents are more likely to recover fully.

Chronic venous insufficiency

28

Aby Mitchell

Figure 28.1 Blood flow. Source: Peate. I. (2021) *Fundamentals of Applied Pathophysiology*, figure 9.1, Wiley.

■ = Oxygenated blood
■ = Deoxygenated blood

- Systemic capillaries of head, neck and upper limbs
- Left pulmonary artery
- Aorta
- Pulmonary capillaries of left lung
- Pulmonary trunk
- Left pulmonary veins
- Superior vena cava
- Left atrium
- Right atrium
- Left ventricle
- Right ventricle
- Inferior vena cava
- Hepatic portal vein
- Systemic capillaries of gastrointestinal tract
- Arterioles
- Venules

Table 28.1 Mechanisms of action.

The heart	The heart exerts as mild 'pull' on the veins due to the pressure gradient between the right atrium (pressure is around 0 mmHg) and the venous system. This is sufficient to produce some blood flow back to the heart when the person is horizontal, but insufficient in aiding venous return when upright.
Veins	Dilate and contract.
The respirator pump	Plays a limited role in venous return. During inspiration the diaphragm pushes against the abdomen, causing a rise in pressure in the intra-abdominal veins. At the same time the pressure in the thorax falls (pressure also falls in the intra thoracic veins and right atrium), blood is drawn from the abdominal cavity into the thorax. The deeper the inspiration the greater venous return.
Calf muscle and foot pumps	These are the most important mechanisms for aiding venous return. The foot pump (contraction of the plantar muscles during movement) squeezes and empties veins in the foot. During exercise, the calf muscle contracts, compressing the deep vein and forcing displacement of blood. The one-way values prevent blood from refluxing, forcing the flow upwards against gravity. When the muscles relax the deep vein expands which causes pressure to drop below that of the superficial veins. The resulting pressure gradient draws blood via the perforator veins from the superficial veins into the deep vein. As exercise continues, muscle contraction squeezes the refilled vein, forcing blood towards the heart. This is a continuous cycle.

Table 28.2 Risk factors for venous insufficiency.

Family history	Some evidence suggests that venous disease is hereditary. Ask patients if any relatives had/have a history of venous disease or oedema.
Previous trauma	Leg injury inclusive of fractures, broken bones, soft tissue injuries, drug use, phlebitis and any other injury that can damage veins, impair mobility or cause DVT.
Previous surgery	Previous surgery to the leg including fractures or flap surgery that cause damage to veins, lymphatics, ankle mobility or gait.
DVT	History of major surgery which may have caused DVT including abdominal surgery or orthopaedic surgery, prolonged immobility. Any clotting disorders, previous long-distance travel, pregnancy and oral contraceptive pill. The effects of DVT can manifest over decades after the event.
Varicose veins	Swollen and enlarged veins are caused by malfunctioning valves.
Mobility	The calf muscle relies on good ankle function to pump blood back to the heart through the veins. Patients with calf muscle wastage due to poor mobility, long-term bandaging, arthritis, and ulcer pain are less likely to reduce venous hypertension through exercise.
Obesity	Obesity of patients who are overweight are more at risk of venous disease. This increases pressure on valves by the increase in hydrostatic pressure (pressure exerted by fluid at rest due to the force of gravity) in veins of the lower extremities and abdomen.
Pregnancy	Pregnancy causes increased abdominal pressure and hormonal changes can affect the muscle layer within veins making them more vulnerable to becoming varicosed.
Age	Increasing age affects patients' mobility find it hard to mobilise particularly if they suffer from other conditions such as arthritis.
Occupation	Jobs which required prolonged sitting and standing appear to increase the risk of venous disease. This is presumed to be due to prolonged pressure in the veins.
Chronic constipation	Chronic constipation increases the amount of pressure on the veins with can lead to valve damage.

The venous system

The venous system is an important part of the circulatory system. The heart may be the principal organ that pumps blood round the body, but it is the vascular system that transports the blood throughout the system. Blood flows through arteries and arterioles transporting oxygen, nutrients, and other substances essential for cellular metabolism and homeostatic regulation. Veins and venules are responsible for carrying deoxygenated (oxygen-depleted) blood towards the heart see Figure 28.1.

The veins have an important job forcing blood upwards towards the heart against gravity. Table 28.1 depicts all the mechanisms of action. Venous disease occurs when the calf muscle and foot muscle pumps are unable to effectively empty veins. This results in venous hypertension (increased pressure in the veins), often due to valve incompetence allowing blood to flow backwards 'reflux' towards capillaries as well as forwards towards the heart. Valve incompetence in the deep veins causes an increased pressure on the valve below and the corresponding perforator vein valve. As a result, these valves also become incompetent causing the superficial veins to varicose and progression of venous disease. The same 'effect' happens whether the primary incompetence occurs in the perforator or superficial veins.

Chronic venous insufficiency

Chronic venous insufficiency (CVI) in the lower limbs is one of the most common conditions in adults in the western world, with a prevalence of between 25 and 40% and 10–20% in women and men respectively. CVI refers to functional changes that occur in the lower limbs due to persistent elevated venous pressures. Commonly the result is venous reflux due to faulty valve function. There are several factors that increase the risk of venous insufficiency; these are identified in Table 28.2.

Classification

Classification of venous insufficiency is difficult due to the broad spectrum of venous complaints which range from minor blemishes to chronic venous ulcers. However, early classification and intervention can have significant results in the prevention of further deterioration and venous leg ulceration. The CEAP system is an internationally accepted standard for describing patients with venous disease.

CEAP

- C – Clinical presentation
- E – Aetiology
- A – Abnormalities found
- P – Pathophysiology of problem encountered

C0

No visible or palpable signs of venous disease. This category is often overlooked – however early intervention at this stage can have excellent results. Patients report tired, heavy legs.

C1

Spider veins are visible, telangiectasis or reticular veins. These are the first visible signs of venous problems.

C2

Significant indicator of CVI. Visible, palpable varicose veins of variable origin – saphenous, accessory saphenous and non-saphenous over 3 mm long. Venous valve damage causes backflow and blood pooling which results in the vein walls stretching beyond repair and makes it increasingly difficult for the venous system to pump back to the heart. Once CVI has transitioned to CEAP C2 classification the delivery of essential nutrients and oxygen to the surrounding tissue is compromised and complications start to develop.

C2r

Recurrent varicose veins.

C3

Pitting oedema mostly found in the ankle which can resolve partially when the patient lies down for a period of time. This is caused by venous blood and protein in the lower extremities. Not to be confused with cardiac or renal oedema.

C4

Changes in skin and subcutaneous tissue secondary to chronic venous disease.

C4a

Hyperpigmentation – a red/brown discolouration of the skin caused by the breakdown and leakage of red blood cells from the capillary networks in the surrounding skin.

C4a

Varicose eczema – caused by irritation of the blood products leaked into the surrounding skin.

C4b

Atrophie blanche – white lacy areas of vascular tissue interspersed by tiny red dots which are caused by engorged capillaries.

C4b

Lipodermatosclerosis – a hardening of the subcutaneous fatty layer caused by leakage and laying down of fibrin from the capillary network.

C4c

Corona phlebectatica (ankle flare) – tiny varicose veins found on the inner aspect of the ankle due to perforator vein incompetence.

C5

Healed leg ulcer. Recurrence rates for healed leg ulcers can be as high as 70%.

C6

Active leg ulcer defined as a break in the skin which has failed to heal in two weeks.

C6r

Recurrent active venous ulcer.

The progression of venous disease to venous leg ulceration is not fully understood. There are several theories as to how this happens, but none are conclusive, and it is thought that it may be a combination of several.

Theories

The fibrin cuff theory

Venous hypertension causes capillary distension which results in endothelial pore dilation, allowing fibrinogen to leak through and lay cuffs along the capillary wall. The fibrin cuffs inhibit oxygen and nutrient transfer into the surrounding tissue and leads to atrophic skin, tissue hypoxia, induration, lipodermatosclerosis (see CEAP classification) and ulceration. In addition, chronic inflammation occurs due to extracellular proteins and leucocytes.

The white blood cell theory

White blood cells adhere (become trapped) to the endothelium of the capillaries as a result of venous hypertension. The accumulation and activation of trapped white blood cells in patients with venous hypertension release toxic metabolites, TNF (tumour necrosis factor – a pro inflammatory cytokine) and proteolytic enzymes which cause vascular destruction and lead to increased vascular permeability. Leucocytes become trapped in the capillaries in static blood and obstruct the flow. Monocytes become active causing skin damage by the release of cytokines. This links onto the fibrin cuff theory as increased permeability leads to fibrin cuff formation.

Mechanical theory

High pressure in the capillary bed leads to oedema which increases tissue pressure and stretches the skin. It is thought that ulceration arises from tissue ischaemia (restriction of the blood supply to the tissue) causing hypoxia and a shortage in glucose required for cellular metabolism.

The 'trap' growth factor theory

Growth factors and inflammatory cells are trapped in the fibrin cuff preventing their normal function in epidermal tissue repair.

CVI is a lifelong condition which requires early assessment and intervention to delay disease progression and reduce the risk of venous leg ulceration. The CEAP tool is a useful guide to assess the level of patient's insufficiency and plan treatment and care.

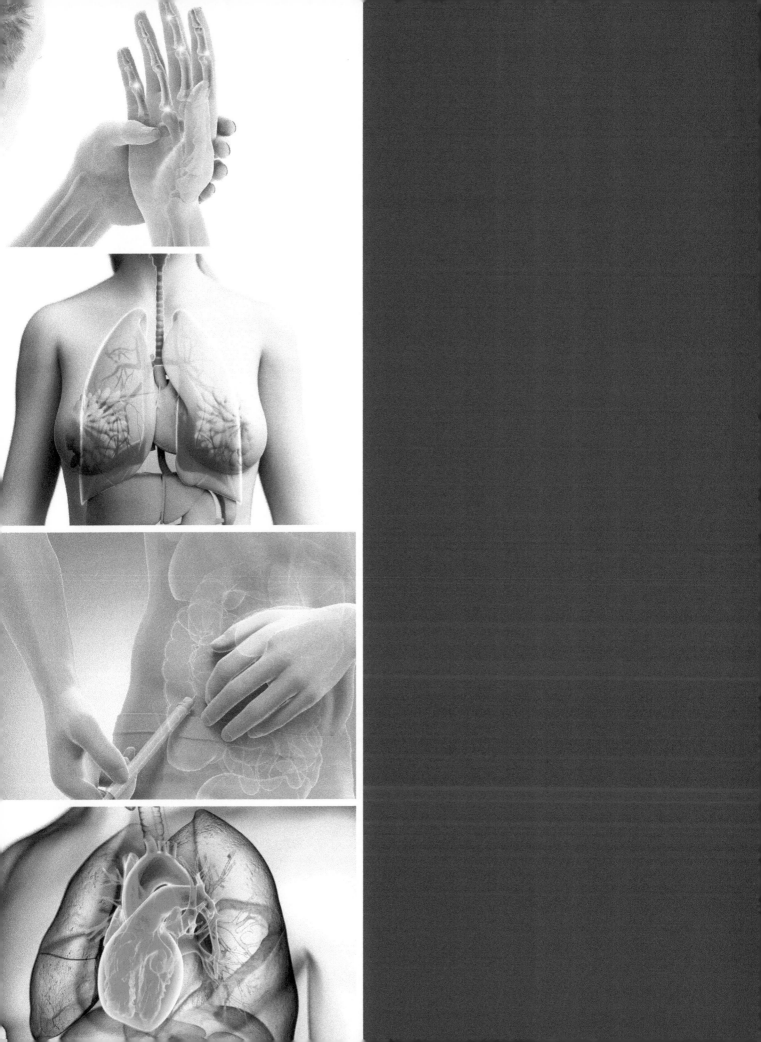

29 Chronic obstructive pulmonary disease (COPD)

Barry Hill

Table 29.1 COPD symptoms.

Suspect COPD in people aged over 35 yr with a risk factor (such as smoking, occupational or environmental exposure) and one or more of the following symptoms:	• Breathlessness – typically persistent, progressive over time, and worse on exertion • Chronic/recurrent cough • Regular sputum production • Frequent lower respiratory tract infections • Wheeze
Other symptoms which may be present include:	• Weight loss, anorexia, and fatigue – common in severe COPD but other causes must be considered • Waking at night with breathlessness • Ankle swelling • Chest pain – uncommon in COPD • Haemoptysis – uncommon in COPD • Reduced exercise tolerance

Table 29.2 Medical Research Council (MRC) dyspnoea scale.

Grade	Level of activity
1	Not troubled by breathlessness except during strenuous exercise
2	Short of breath when hurrying or walking up a slight hill
3	Walks slower than contemporaries on the level because of breathlessness, or must stop for breath when walking at own pace
4	Stops for breath after walking about 100 m or after a few minutes on the level
5	Too breathless to leave the house, or breathless when dressing or undressing

Figures 29.1 Emphysema. Source: COPD for Dummies. Wiley. Chapter 1, p.13.

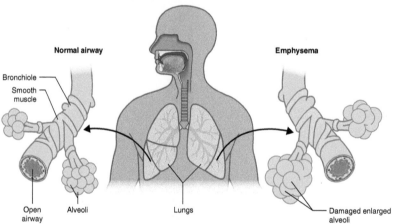

Figure 29.2 Bronchitis. Source: Felner, K. Schneider, M. (2008) COPD for Dummies. Wiley. Chapter 1, p.12.

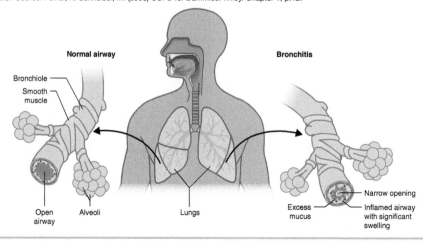

Introduction

The Global Initiative for Chronic Obstructive Lung Disease (GOLD) (2022) define chronic obstructive pulmonary disease (COPD) as a preventable and treatable disease state characterised by airflow limitation that is not fully reversible. It encompasses both emphysema and chronic bronchitis. The airflow limitation is usually progressive and is associated with an abnormal inflammatory response of the lungs to noxious particles or gases. It is primarily caused by cigarette smoking. Although COPD affects the lungs, it also has significant systemic consequences. Exacerbations and co-morbidities are important contributors to the overall condition and prognosis in individual patients. An estimated 1.2 million people are living with diagnosed COPD – considerably more than the 835 000 estimated by the Department of Health in 2011. In terms of diagnosed cases, this makes COPD the second most common lung disease in the UK, after asthma. Around 2% of the whole population – 4.5% of all people aged over 40 years – live with diagnosed COPD.

Pathophysiology

Typical pathophysiology of COPD is an amalgamation of emphysema and chronic bronchitis.

Emphysema

Emphysema is the permanent enlargement of the airspaces beyond the terminal bronchiole and the destruction of the elastic recoil of the alveolar wall. This degeneration of lung tissue is thought to be related to the action of destructive enzymes called proteases. Proteases are released from neutrophils and macrophages during respiratory infections. To minimise the effects of proteases, lung tissue produces a substance called α1-antitrypsin, which counteracts the destructive action of protease. Individuals with emphysema produce less effective α1-antitrypsin and alveolar destruction is allowed to continue unabated. This reduction in the efficacy of α1-antitrypsin is predominantly caused by smoking. The resultant damaged alveoli lack the elastic recoil that is required for exhalation, often resulting in over-inflation and air trapping. Increased intrathoracic pressure pushes the diaphragm downwards, disturbing its natural concave shape and making breathing difficult. Respiratory infections can easily develop as individuals find it increasingly difficult to expectorate secretions. Also, further destruction of the alveolar walls and nearby capillaries results in reduced surface area for external respiration, rendering the patient at risk of hypoxaemia and hypoxia. See Figure 29.1.

Chronic bronchitis

Chronic bronchitis is defined as the presence of a productive cough lasting for three months in each of two consecutive years when other pulmonary and cardiac causes of cough have been ruled out. Chronic bronchitis is characterised by increased mucus production and damaged bronchial cilia in the bronchi. The increase in mucus stimulates airway irritant receptors, resulting in a chronic cough. Constant airway irritation produces inflammation and a thickening of the bronchial wall, and the destruction of cilia makes mucus clearance difficult, and mucus collects and blocks the smaller airways as a result. The individual is then susceptible to further infections which cause yet more irritation and inflammation. Over time, increasing numbers of airways become blocked, reducing external respiration. The increased mucus production and cilia dysfunction found in chronic bronchitis occurs in response to a constant bombardment of inhaled pollutants such as cigarette smoke. See Figure 29.2.

Pathophysiology of exacerbation of COPD

Exacerbations are often associated with increased neutrophilic inflammation and, in some mild exacerbations, increased numbers of eosinophils. Exacerbations can be caused by infection (bacterial or viral), air pollution, and changes in ambient temperature. In mild exacerbations, airflow obstruction is unchanged or only slightly increased. Severe exacerbations are associated with worsening of pulmonary gas exchange due to increased inequality between ventilation and perfusion and subsequent respiratory muscle fatigue. The worsening ventilation–perfusion relation results from airway inflammation, oedema, mucous hypersecretion, and bronchoconstriction. These reduce ventilation and cause hypoxic vasoconstriction of pulmonary arterioles, which in turn impairs perfusion. Respiratory muscle fatigue and alveolar hypoventilation can contribute to hypoxaemia, hypercapnia, and respiratory acidosis, and lead to severe respiratory failure and death. Hypoxia and respiratory acidosis can induce pulmonary vasoconstriction, which increases the load on the right ventricle and, together with renal and hormonal changes, results in peripheral oedema.

Symptoms

COPD imposes a substantial burden on individuals with the disease, which can include a range of symptoms (Table 29.1). COPD is associated with a significant socio-economic burden, which is predicted to increase over the coming decades. A range of symptoms and their impact on patients define the daily burden of COPD borne by an individual. The most common symptoms of COPD are dyspnoea (Table 29.2), cough, and sputum production, and less common but troublesome symptoms are wheezing, chest tightness, and chest congestion. However, reported frequencies differ depending on the patient population and severity of disease. For example, cough has been reported as the most common symptom in patients with mild COPD.

Causes

Tobacco smoke is a key factor in the development and progression of COPD. Exposure to air pollutants in the home and workplace, genetic factors, and respiratory infections also play a role. People should try to avoid inhaling tobacco smoke, home and workplace air pollutants, and respiratory infections to prevent developing COPD. Early detection of COPD may change its course and progress.

Coronary artery Disease

30

Sadie Diamond-Fox

Figure 30.1 Risk factors and manifestations of cardiovascular disease. Source: Aaronson et al. (2012), p. 76.

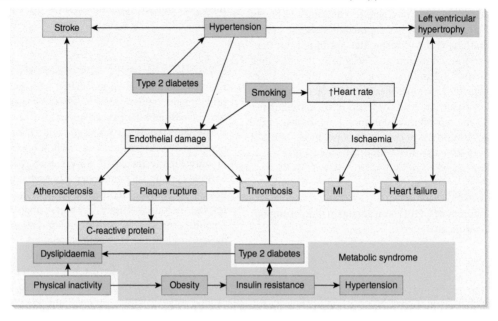

Figure 30.2 Pathophysiology of atherosclerosis and subsequent plaque rupture. (a) Normal coronary artery structure. (b)–(d) CAD Steps 1–3. Source: England, T. and Nasim, A. (eds.) (2014). *ABC of Arterial and Venous Disease: ABC of Arterial and Venous Disease*, 3e, Wiley.

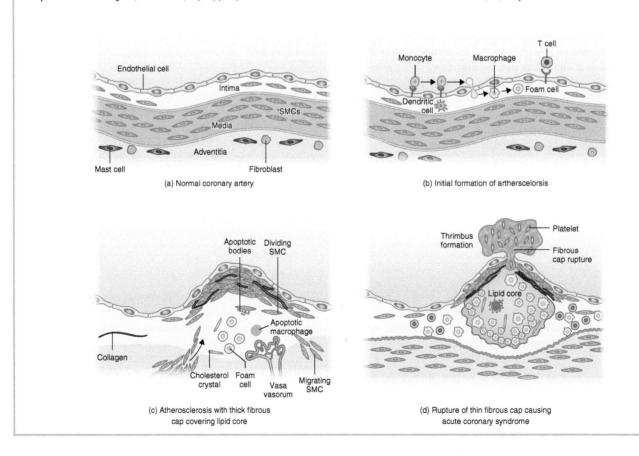

(a) Normal coronary artery

(b) Initial formation of artherscelorsis

(c) Atherosclerosis with thick fibrous cap covering lipid core

(d) Rupture of thin fibrous cap causing acute coronary syndrome

Definition and epidemiology

Coronary artery disease (CAD) is also known as coronary heart disease (CHD) and is one of the most common heart conditions globally. It can lead to a plethora of complications including, but not limited to; ischaemic heart disease, heart failure, acute coronary syndromes and arrhythmias. CAD is one of the 'five big killers' in the United Kingdom (UK) alongside liver disease, respiratory disease, stroke and cancer. According to the Primary Care Mortality Database (PCMD), mortality rates from CAD continue to remain high and despite rapid advances in healthcare provision, remains a major cause of premature death in the UK. It remains one of leading causes of death worldwide and is estimated to represent 2.2% of the overall global disease burden.

A seminal multigenerational study (The Framingham Heart Study) that began in 1948, and continues to this day, has shaped the way in which we provide health care for this patient group globally through the gathering of data from over 14000 participants. The Framingham Heart Study has identified several risk factors for the development of CAD and the associated manifestations of cardiovascular disease (Figure 30.1).

Risk factors can be classified in to modifiable (smoking, hyperlipidaemia, hypertension, diabetes mellitus, obesity, and physical inactivity) and non-modifiable (genetic predisposition, age and gender). There are several screening programmes that exist internationally to monitor for the development of cardiovascular diseases.

Pathogenesis

CAD involves the formation of atherosclerotic plaques within the coronary artery lumen. Normal coronary artery structure (Figure 30.2a) contains three layers: intima (inner most layer), media and adventitia (outermost layer). The intima is lined by a layer of endothelial cells which are in contact with the blood, and smooth muscle cells (SMC) which are located within the intima. Endothelial cells are the site of much interest when establishing the reason for the development of multiple vascular pathologies due to their role in haemostasis, angiogenesis (formation of new blood vessels) and regulation of vascular tone (vasodilation and vasoconstriction). They can respond to inflammatory stimuli by expression of various cell membrane receptors which control immune cell recruitment.

SMCs are also present in the vessel media and are embedded in a complex extracellular matrix which contains collagen and elastin. Finally, the adventitia contains inactivated immune cells called fibroblasts and mast cells. Each of these vessel layers and their resident cells play a role in the pathogenesis of atherosclerosis and subsequent CAD.

Atherosclerosis is a chronic inflammatory disorder that accompanies the ageing process. The pathogenesis of atherosclerosis and subsequent CAD is complex, but can be simplified into the following steps:

STEP 1 (Figure 30.2b)

a Lipids (low density lipoproteins [LDL]) accumulate in the intimal space of the artery wall to form a fatty streak. This fatty streak formation begins in the first decade of life and can be accelerated by the modifiable and non-modifiable cardiovascular risk factors.

b Activated endothelial cells subjected to stimulus (hyperlipidaemia, hypertension, inflammation) express adhesion molecules to which inflammatory cells (monocytes) bind.

c Monocytes are then able to migrate into the intima of the coronary vessel wall and differentiate into macrophages.

d Activated macrophages ingest LDL to form foam cells.

STEP 2 (Figure 30.2c)

a Vascular smooth muscle cell (VSMC) migration – Cytokines and growth factor released from foam cells cause smooth muscle cell migration from the media into the intima of the coronary vessel wall. VSMCs change from a contractile phenotype to a 'repair/synthetic' phenotype, which has been shown to be an important factor in the formation of micro vessels within the vessel intima due to their ability to promote development and growth of collateral blood vessels via arteriogenesis. VSMC phenotype switching has been shown to play an important role in the advancement of atherosclerosis and subsequent complications of plague rupture.

b The extra-cellular matrix present within the vessel intima begins to produce/synthesise collagen and elastin, both of which promote atherosclerotic plaque stability through the formation of a fibrous 'cap', but can also contribute to coronary artery stenosis, further increasing the mismatch between oxygen delivery and oxygen demand to the heart.

c Over time, the plaque may become 'stable' and become calcified, if no further insults occur to the vascular endothelium.

STEP 3 (Figure 30.2d)

a In an unstable plaque, the endothelium continues to be activated, foam cells continue to be formed and enter a cycle of apoptosis (programmed cell death) and release their LDL contents into the vessel intima which then form a lipid core.

b SMC continue to secrete extracellular matrix molecules that further entrap LDL particles.

c As the necrotic fibrous plaque core increases, the fibrous cap may become thinner (VSMC phenotype switching may also be implicated here). This renders the cap vulnerable to rupture.

d Plaque rupture triggers platelet activation, resulting thrombus formation and acute coronary syndrome.

Symptoms

Symptoms of CAD depend upon the extent of coronary artery damage. Severe damage results in disrupted blood flow to the myocardium. The disruption of blood flows results in an imbalance between oxygen supply and demand and can eventually lead to angina (Chapter 20), shortness of breath and myocardial infarction.

Recommendations for clinical practice

Evidence-based guidelines advocate risk assessment of patients with suspected CAD. Scoring tools such as the QRISK3 and/or CAD Score system may be utilised. The promotion of risk reduction via treatment of modifiable risk factors, such as lifestyle modification including smoking cessation and weight management, and screening for those with non-modifiable/fixed risk factors. Institution of preventive pharmacological therapy where appropriate is also recommended, such as lipid modification therapy.

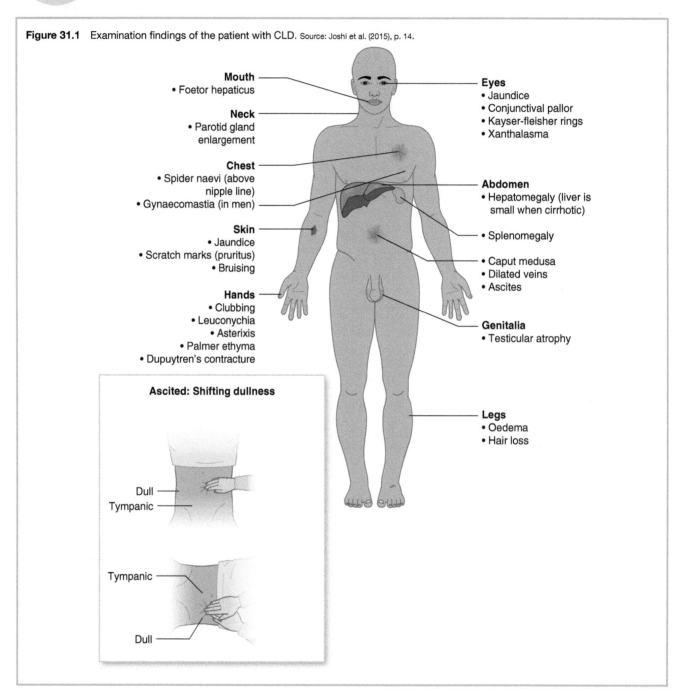

Chronic liver disease

Sadie Diamond-Fox

31

Figure 31.1 Examination findings of the patient with CLD. Source: Joshi et al. (2015), p. 14.

Mouth
• Foetor hepaticus

Neck
• Parotid gland enlargement

Chest
• Spider naevi (above nipple line)
• Gynaecomastia (in men)

Skin
• Jaundice
• Scratch marks (pruritus)
• Bruising

Hands
• Clubbing
• Leuconychia
• Asterixis
• Palmer ethyma
• Dupuytren's contracture

Eyes
• Jaundice
• Conjunctival pallor
• Kayser-fleisher rings
• Xanthalasma

Abdomen
• Hepatomegaly (liver is small when cirrhotic)
• Splenomegaly
• Caput medusa
• Dilated veins
• Ascites

Genitalia
• Testicular atrophy

Legs
• Oedema
• Hair loss

Ascited: Shifting dullness

Dull
Tympanic

Tympanic

Dull

Long-term Conditions in Adults at a Glance, First Edition. Edited by Aby Mitchell, Barry Hill, and Ian Peate.
© 2023 John Wiley & Sons Ltd. Published 2023 by John Wiley & Sons Ltd.

Definition and statistics

Chronic liver disease (CLD) encompasses of spectrum of diseases that cause a progressive cycle of inflammation destruction and regeneration of the liver parenchyma, over a period of greater than six months. CLD remains a national public health concern, despite rapid advances in health-care provision. Liver disease (known as of the 'five big killers') is the third leading cause of premature death in the UK, with a continued exponential rise in standardised UK mortality rate much greater than heart disease, respiratory disease, stroke and cancer. A concerning dataset released annually shows that the number of deaths occurring within the UK due to unspecified hepatitis, fibrosis and cirrhosis of the liver in the UK continues to rise.

There are a number of known risk factors for the development of cirrhosis, these include chronic alcohol misuse (CAM) (defined as consuming more than 14 units alcohol/week on a regular basis), obesity and type 2 diabetes (T2DM). CAM, obesity and T2DM are known to promote fatty infiltration into the liver (steatosis) which plays a major role in the pathogenesis of CLD. Non-alcoholic fatty liver disease (NAFLD)/non-alcoholic steatohepatitis (NASH), chronic viral hepatitis (B, C, variants), autoimmune disease such as primary sclerosing cholangitis and autoimmune hepatitis and genetic causes such as Wilson's disease, alpha-1 antitrypsin deficiency and hereditary haemochromatosis are all causes of CLD.

Pathogenesis

The pathogenesis of CLD is commonly classified into four stages:

1 Hepatitis (also known as steatosis)
2 Fibrosis
3 Cirrhosis
4 Hepatocellular carcinoma (HCC).

The liver is integral to multiple homeostatic mechanisms within the body, including but not limited to; excretion of bile, synthesis of clotting factors and proteins, detoxification of harmful products of metabolism and xenobiotics (e.g. drugs) and breakdown of red blood cells. The pathogenesis of CLD is an insidious, chronic inflammatory disorder which leads to cyclical damage to hepatocytes, destruction of the liver parenchyma and regeneration and eventual fibrosis and cirrhosis. Continuation of the inflammatory insult can lead to eventual necrosis and apoptosis of hepatocytes and can ultimately lead to rapid decompensation and activation of malignant pathologies within the liver itself, or as a metastatic variance. Not only is the parenchymal architecture of the liver disrupted, but vascular reorganisation also occurs.

Symptoms

There are multiple signs and symptoms of CLD (Figure 31.1). CLD may present with non-specific symptoms such as weight loss and fatigue. Due to its insidious nature and the liver's ability to compensate, the pathogenesis of CLD can occur relatively silently with minimal systemic or even laboratory signs of disease. However, it is often not until an acute event (e.g. infection, increased alcohol consumption, surgery) presents itself that patients with CLD discover the extent of the underlying damage. The acute event causes increased demand upon an already challenged system which has little to no reserve. This can lead to an acute decompensated state which may have life-threatening sequelae, such as oesophageal varices rupture, hepatic encephalopathy, spontaneous bacterial peritonitis and hepatorenal syndrome.

More than 90% of patients with cirrhosis develop portal hypertension (PH) secondary to intrahepatic architectural changes, activated stellate and vascular smooth-muscle cells of the intrahepatic veins and active contraction of myofibroblasts. PH involves portosystemic shunting of blood due to an increase in vascular resistance to the portal blood flow secondary to pre-hepatic, intrahepatic or posthepatic causes. The presence of telangiectasia and spider angioma accompanied with jaundice are highly suggestive of PH.

Jaundice is a direct result of hyperbilirubinemia and associated deposition of bile pigments in tissue rich elastin, which can be classified into pre-hepatic/unconjugated/haemolytic, hepatic/hepatocellular and post-hepatic/cholestatic causes. Haemolytic causes of jaundice are relatively uncommon and distinguishing between hepatocellular and cholestatic causes is the most common differentiation required in clinical practice. Hepatocellular jaundice (HCJ) refers to diffuse damage to the liver parenchyma, resulting in an inability of bilirubin transportation across the hepatocyte into the bile. This can occur at any point between uptake of unconjugated bilirubin into the hepatocyte, to the transport of conjugated bilirubin into the biliary canaliculi. Cholestatic jaundice may be caused by: failure of hepatocytes to initiate bile flow; obstruction within the bile ducts, or obstruction of outflow into the extra-hepatic ducts.

Recommendations for clinical practice

Evidence-based guidelines advocate the immediate blood serum assays for several tests in all patients with clinical evidence of cirrhosis, regardless of aetiology. These tests include prothrombin time (PT) to determine abnormalities in plasma concentrations of vitamin K dependent factors of both the extrinsic and common coagulation pathway (factors VII, X, V, pro-thrombin and fibrinogen) which is determinant of severity of disease. Aspartate aminotransferase (AST), alanine aminotransferase (ALT) and total bilirubin assays are also strongly recommended. These tests can aid in the differentiation of where damage may be taking place and, depending on the pattern of elevation, can inform differential diagnoses. Consideration to investigations such as viral serology, iron, ferritin, copper, autoantibodies, serum ceruloplasmin and alpha one antitrypsin should be given. A liver Doppler ultrasound, computer tomography (CT) scan, liver biopsy and transient elastography may also need to be performed.

The use of the Child–Pugh scoring system, Model for End-Stage Liver Disease (MELD) and the United Kingdom Model for End-Stage Liver Disease (UKELD) are evidence-based scoring systems for quantifying the severity of CLD and stratifying those that may require transplantation.

As with any health-care intervention, it is important to employ a holistic approach and the management of CLD is no exception. Patients require robust education strategies in order to empower them to prevent further damage. Such interventions include: avoidance of alcohol; healthy eating and exercise regimens; screening for viral hepatitis (B & C) and vaccination against hepatitis A & B; and safe utilisation of over the counter drugs (paracetamol). Both patients and health-care professionals, particularly registered prescribers, may find the LIVERTOX® database (http://www.livertox.nih.gov) useful when considering pharmaceutical interventions when caring for the patient with CLD.

32 Depression

Sarah Bisp and Louise Lingwood

Figure 32.1 Considerations for health and social-care professionals.

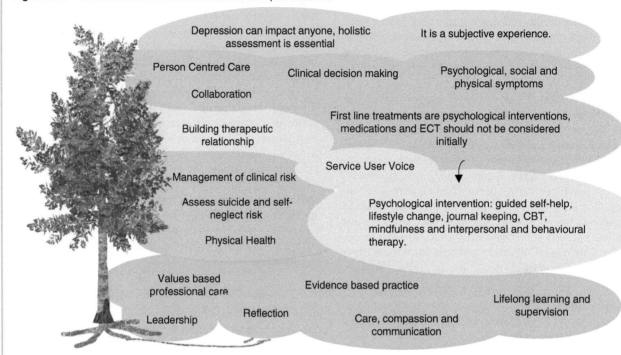

- Depression can impact anyone, holistic assessment is essential
- It is a subjective experience.
- Person Centred Care
- Clinical decision making
- Psychological, social and physical symptoms
- Collaboration
- Building therapeutic relationship
- First line treatments are psychological interventions, medications and ECT should not be considered initially
- Service User Voice
- Management of clinical risk
- Assess suicide and self-neglect risk
- Psychological intervention: guided self-help, lifestyle change, journal keeping, CBT, mindfulness and interpersonal and behavioural therapy.
- Physical Health
- Values based professional care
- Evidence based practice
- Lifelong learning and supervision
- Leadership
- Reflection
- Care, compassion and communication

Figure 32.2 Types of depression.

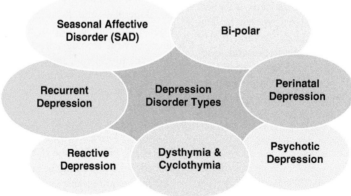

Seasonal Affective Disorder is sometimes known as winter depression as the symptoms worsen in the colder, darker months. Symptoms may include persistent low mood, low energy, guilt, worthlessness, craving carbohydrates, poor concentration.

Bi-polar Disorder is characterised by energetic highs (mania) and the extreme lows of depression. These mood swings can last for several weeks or months. Patterns may include rapid changes in mood or a mixed state or high energy and very low mood.

Recurrent Depression is repeated depression that comes and goes over a period leaving people feeling unmotivated and drained. During the times in between a person's mood may stabilise, and functioning improves.

Perinatal Depression is present if depression is present whilst pregnant (anti-natal) or during the year following birth (Post-natal). Baby blues can happen briefly in the first 10 days following birth due to the changes having a new baby brings. Post-natal depression is longer term and symptoms may be mild or severe.

Depression Disorder Types: Seasonal Affective Disorder (SAD), Bi-polar, Recurrent Depression, Perinatal Depression, Reactive Depression, Dysthymia & Cyclothymia, Psychotic Depression

Reactive Depression describes symptoms of depression that occur due to a challenging situation, stressor or external problem. It is also known as situational depression

Dysthymia is also known as persistent depressive disorder and is milder but long lasting than recurrent depression. It can be characterised by episodes of severe depression at times. It is linked to chronic stress or trauma along with environmental, psychological and genetic factors. Cyclothymia relates to unstable moods and is more commonly associated with **bi-polar**.

Psychotic Depression is a subtype of major depression (differentiated from schizophrenia – chapter 47) that includes a psychotic episode. The psychosis may include hallucinations (sensory perception such as hearing voices) and/or delusions (intense false beliefs that persist despite evidence.

What is depression?

Sadness is a normal response to difficult or upsetting situations particularly in the context of bereavement or chronic physical health. However, when feelings of sadness become difficult to control, are intense, pervasive and prevent individuals from participating in daily activities, this may be a sign of depression. Untreated depressive disorders can become chronic in nature and associated with a negative course and outcome. Health and social care professionals work across a variety of settings and will encounter people with clinical depression. All health and social care professionals have a role to play in the prevention, assessment, diagnosis and the management of depression (Figure 32.1).

Depressive disorders

Depressive disorders are forms of mood disorders and include recurrent depression, reactive depression, dysthymia, cyclothymia, seasonal affective disorder, bi-polar and severe depression with psychotic symptoms (Figure 32.2). Depression can affect anyone at any age. It is believed one in six people report the experience of depression or anxiety in any given week in the UK although this figure is thought to have escalated due to the COVID-19 pandemic.

Clinical features

People with depression can experience a range of symptoms that are cognitive, behavioural and biological in nature dependent on the type of depression experienced (Figure 32.2). Thought content is often negative in nature about the self, the world and the future. Biological symptoms include sleep disturbance, appetite change and loss of libido. Motor activity can increase or decrease and movement and or speech may be affected. Depression is often comorbid with anxiety disorder (Chapter 21) and may be masked by severe anxiety disorder or present as difficulties with anger. The predominant symptom of depression is a pervasive lowering of mood although this is not needed for a diagnosis to be made.

ICD–10 classifies clinically important depressive episodes as mild, moderate and severe based on the number, type and severity of symptoms present and degree of functional impairment. These include low mood, decreased energy and anhedonia (loss of enjoyment in activities once found pleasurable). Other symptoms include: sleep disturbance, irritability and restlessness, inability to concentrate, physical tension, ideas of worthlessness and/or guilt, thoughts of self-harm or death, and low self-esteem.

The severity of the depression (mild, moderate, or severe) depends on several factors including the number of symptoms present, the degree of distress experienced, and interference with daily activities and functioning. Psychotic episodes may be present in severe depression. In some cases, alcohol or substance withdrawal may mimic depressive disorder.

Aetiology

Changes in hormones and chemicals in the body may cause depression. For example, low levels of vitamin B_{12}, thyroid problems or premenstrual syndrome.

A neurotransmitter is a chemical substance that is released at the end of a nerve fibre when triggered by a nerve impulse. They diffuse across the synapse and effects the transfer of the impulse to the next neurone or a target cell. Monoamine neurotransmitter (serotonin and noradrenaline) availability in the synaptic cleft is reduced in depression. Anti-depressant medication acts to increase monoamine availability. Stimulation of the subgenual cingulate cortex deep in the cerebral cortex in the brain also increases monoamine readiness. Exposure to stressful events leads to increased cortisol. Hypercortisolaemia (this can be associated with Cushing disease) has been found in people with severe depression. Hypocortisolaemia (this can be associated with Addison's disease) is linked to symptoms of low mood and atypical depression. Dysfunctional changes to the limbic system and prefrontal cortex (responsible for reward, emotional regulation, and executive function) in the brain have been implicated in depression.

Management

It is important that the depressive disorder is identified through holistic assessment including history, presence of a chronic physical health issue, relationships, social situation, family history, domestic violence and employment. Risks associated with self-neglect and suicide should always be assessed. Psychiatric referral is indicated where depression is severe, bi-polar, recurrent or unresponsive to initial treatments and where suicide risk is present.

Treatment guidance recommend evidence-based psychological interventions as the first line of treatment in preference to pharmacological intervention. Psychoeducation should be offered, and the presentation monitored, and the individual should be referred on for specialist assessment where necessary. Other psychological treatments recommended include cognitive behaviour therapy, interpersonal therapy, mindfulness, and behavioural therapy.

Risk management is essential in the delivery of any psychological intervention and the establishment of a therapeutic relationship is crucial to the delivery of safe, person-centred and high-quality care.

Reservations about pharmacological treatment for depressive disorders exist, not least due to the potential adverse side-effects but also risks related to type 2 diabetes mellitus, serotonin syndrome, hyponatraemia, and an increase in suicidal thoughts. Health-care professionals play a vital role in supporting people with depression to help understand the benefits associated with pharmacological interventions and support them to balance these with the associated risks. Continuing anti-depressant therapy for at least six months may reduce relapse. Anti-depressant discontinuation should be tapered to avoid withdrawal symptoms. In bi-polar, mood stabilisers such as lithium are used (often alongside psychological therapies such as cognitive behavioural therapy (CBT) and mindfulness). Electroconvulsive therapy is used and found effective in cases of severe depression. A healthy lifestyle, active lifestyle and a balanced diet is beneficial.

33 Diabetes mellitus type 1

Charlotte Gordon

Table 33.1 Insulin therapies (Joint Formulary Committee 2023).

Regimen	Description	Indication
Multiple daily injection (MDI) basal bolus regimen	One or more separate daily injections of intermediate or long-acting insulin analogue as the basal (background) insulin alongside multiple bolus injections of short acting insulin before meals. This is a flexible regimen tailored to carbohydrate intake.	This is the first line choice.
Mixed (biphasic) regimen	One, two or three insulin injections per day of intermediate mixed with short acting insulin. The preparation may be mixed by the patient, or a pre-mixed product used.	Use if MDI basal bolus regimen is not possible.
Continuous subcutaneous insulin infusion (CSII) – insulin pump	A regular or continuous amount of insulin – usually rapid acting, delivered by a programmable pump comprising an insulin storage reservoir via a subcutaneous needle or cannula.	Should only be offered to adults who experience disabling hypoglycaemia whilst attempting to achieve their target HbA1c, or who have high HbA1c despite a high level of care. Children, should be offered CSII if MDI is not appropriate.

Figure 33.1 How insulin works. Source: Kelly, S., Wijesundare, S., Webb, J., Mutandwa, Al. and Gordon, C. (2019) *Starting Injectable Treatments in Adults with Type 2 Diabetes*. 3rd Edition. London: Royal College of Nursing.

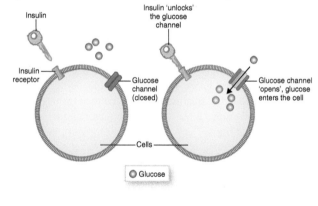

Figure 33.2 Regulation of blood glucose control. Source: Boore J., Cook N. and Shepherd A. (2018) *Essentials of Anatomy and Physiology for Nursing Practice*. London: Sage.

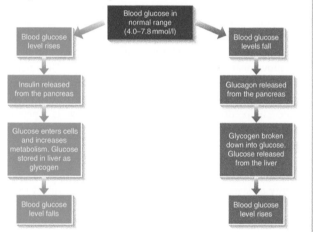

Definition and epidemiology

Type 1 (T1D) and type 2 (T2D) are the two main types of diabetes mellitus alongside gestational diabetes and rarer subtypes of the condition; onset of T1D is most common in childhood and early adulthood. T1DM represents approximately 8–10% of all cases globally, 50% of which occur in adulthood. 84% of people living with T1DM are adults, incidence has steadily increased over the last century at a rate of approximately 2% per year.

T1D is characterised as a complete or relative absolute absence of insulin, resulting in elevated blood glucose levels (hyperglycaemia). Insulin, produced by the Islet of Langerhans within the beta cells of the pancreas, is essential for metabolic functioning; regulating blood glucose levels by facilitating the uptake of glucose by the cells where it can be utilised for energy (Figure 33.1). Insulin is the only hormone which can lower and regulate blood glucose levels. Figure 33.2 details normal blood glucose regulation.

Altered pathophysiology

The pathogenesis of T1D is complex, arising as a result of an autoimmune, T-cell mediated attack of insulin producing cells of the pancreas. In addition, environmental factors, the microbiome, metabolism, and the genome also play a role in the development of the condition. Individuals may present with rapid onset of elevated blood glucose and in some cases, ketoacidosis may be the first sign of T1D (Box 33.1). In some instances, onset may be preceded by infection or other stress, initiating the immune mediated response and beta cell destruction. T1D is not yet preventable. An overview of the pathophysiology is provided in Figure 33.3.

Diagnosis

Initial diagnosis of T1D should be made on clinical grounds in adults presenting with hyperglycaemia (fasting plasma glucose ≥ 7.0 mmol/l, random blood glucose ≥ 11.1 mmol/l or

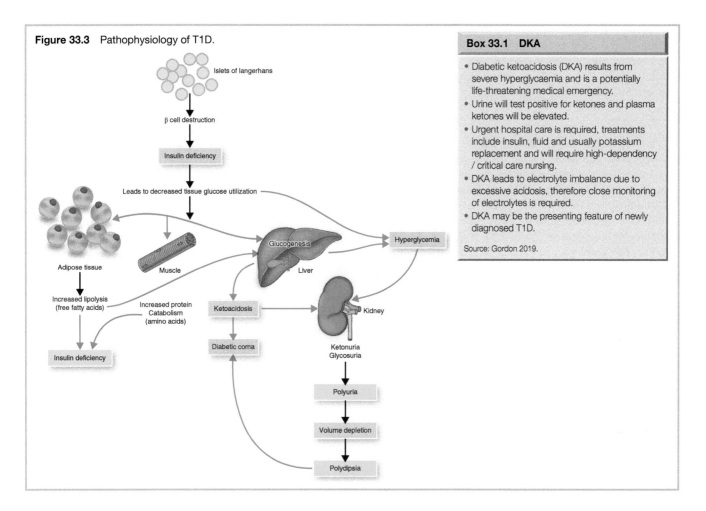

Figure 33.3 Pathophysiology of T1D.

Box 33.1 DKA

- Diabetic ketoacidosis (DKA) results from severe hyperglycaemia and is a potentially life-threatening medical emergency.
- Urine will test positive for ketones and plasma ketones will be elevated.
- Urgent hospital care is required, treatments include insulin, fluid and usually potassium replacement and will require high-dependency / critical care nursing.
- DKA leads to electrolyte imbalance due to excessive acidosis, therefore close monitoring of electrolytes is required.
- DKA may be the presenting feature of newly diagnosed T1D.

HbA1c ≥ 6.5% / 48 mmol/mol). People with T1D may also (but not always) have one or more of the following:
- Ketosis
- Rapid weight loss
- Age of onset under 50 years
- BMI below 25 kg/m² – BMI should not be used alone to diagnose or exclude T1D
- Personal and/or family history of autoimmune disease.
  Presenting symptoms may also include:
- Polydipsia (increased thirst)
- Polyphagia (increased appetite)
- Polyuria (increased urine production)
- Fatigue.

Clinical management

The primary goal of therapy is to maintain blood glucose as near to the normal range as possible without causing unacceptable amounts of hypoglycaemia (low blood glucose).

Upon diagnosis, replacement insulin must be commenced immediately; all people with T1D require insulin therapy. A number of regimens (Table 33.1) are available which usually involve self-injecting multiple daily doses, adjusted to food intake, intended physical activity and current blood glucose levels. The dosage of insulin is determined on an individual basis with regard to blood-glucose concentrations. Hypoglycaemia is an inevitable adverse effect of insulin treatment.

Hypoglycaemia is defined as a random plasma glucose of less than 4 mmol/l and may arise as a result of inadvertent insulin overdose, missed or inadequate meals, unexpected exercise, or an error in the timing of the dose. Treatment for mild to

moderate hypoglycaemia is 10–20 g oral glucose (4–5 jelly babies, 3 sugar lumps, 100 ml Coca-Cola). Severe hypoglycaemia will require glucagon injection which increases plasma glucose by mobilising glycogen from the liver. Frequent low blood glucose can lead to impaired awareness of hypoglycaemia (IAH), whereby the ability to perceive the onset of hypoglycaemia is reduced or absent; in order to restore symptom awareness of hypoglycaemia, recurrent episodes of low blood glucose should be avoided.

HbA1c (glycated haemoglobin) is the recommended means of assessing blood glucose control over an extended period of time (preceding 12 weeks). Elevated HbA1c is associated with an increased risk of diabetes-related complications. HbA1c should be measured every three to six months and targets individualised to consider social factors, risk of complications, comorbidities, and history of hypoglycaemia. Support should be offered to achieve a target of 48 mmol/mol or lower where possible.

Self-monitoring of capillary blood glucose ('finger prick testing') provides information on the effectiveness of glucose metabolism and guides interventions for optimal control. Blood glucose levels should be measured at least 4 times per day (before each meal and before bed); additional testing may be required if target HbA1c levels are not met, when experiencing hypoglycaemia, during illness, before during and after sport, when planning pregnancy or when there is a legal requirement, such as before driving. Adults should aim for a fasting plasma glucose level of 5–7 mmol/l on waking, 4–7 mmol/l before meals at other times of the day and 5–9 mmol/l 90 minutes after eating.

Continuous glucose monitoring (CGM) is now offered to all people with T1D. A CGM, wearable device, continuously measures subcutaneous blood glucose levels sending the readings to a display device or smartphone, significantly reducing the need for finger-prick testing. A number of devices are available with various functionality including hypo/hyperglycaemic alarms, trend arrows and real time glucose data which can enhance clinical care. CGM has been consistently demonstrated to improve HbA1c.

Other clinical considerations

T1D demands significant levels of self-management and structured education is integral to diabetes care and self-management. Education programmes can enable people with T1D to match their insulin doses to their food choice (carbohydrate counting) whilst keeping blood glucose levels within normal ranges. Education programmes should promote insight into healthy eating alongside developing knowledge to adjust insulin doses to reduce glucose excursions when varying dietary intake.

In addition, people with T1D should be encouraged to engage in physical activity, receiving education to understand the effects of exercise on blood glucose levels and required insulin dosage adjustments. Physical activity reduces cardiovascular risk factors, enhances well-being, and improves insulin sensitivity.

Complications

Despite the differing pathophysiology of T1D, T2D, and other subtypes of diabetes, the resulting complications are the same. Continued elevation of blood glucose levels can lead to progressive macro and microvascular damage. Long-term complications are serious and include accelerated atherosclerosis, retinopathy, neuropathy, nephropathy, and sexual dysfunction. Diabetes is the most common cause of:

- Blindness in working aged people
- End-stage renal failure
- Non-traumatic lower limb amputation due to neuropathy and peripheral vascular disease.

In addition, alongside physical complications, the condition can significantly impact emotional well-being resulting in 'diabetes distress' or major depressive disorders.

Diabetes and its complications account for 11.3% all-cause mortality in adults aged 20–79 in 2019 and nearly 50% of these are less than 60 years of age. Highlighting the importance of effective management and prevention of complications. Early detection and management of complications can often prevent disability and improve quality of life.

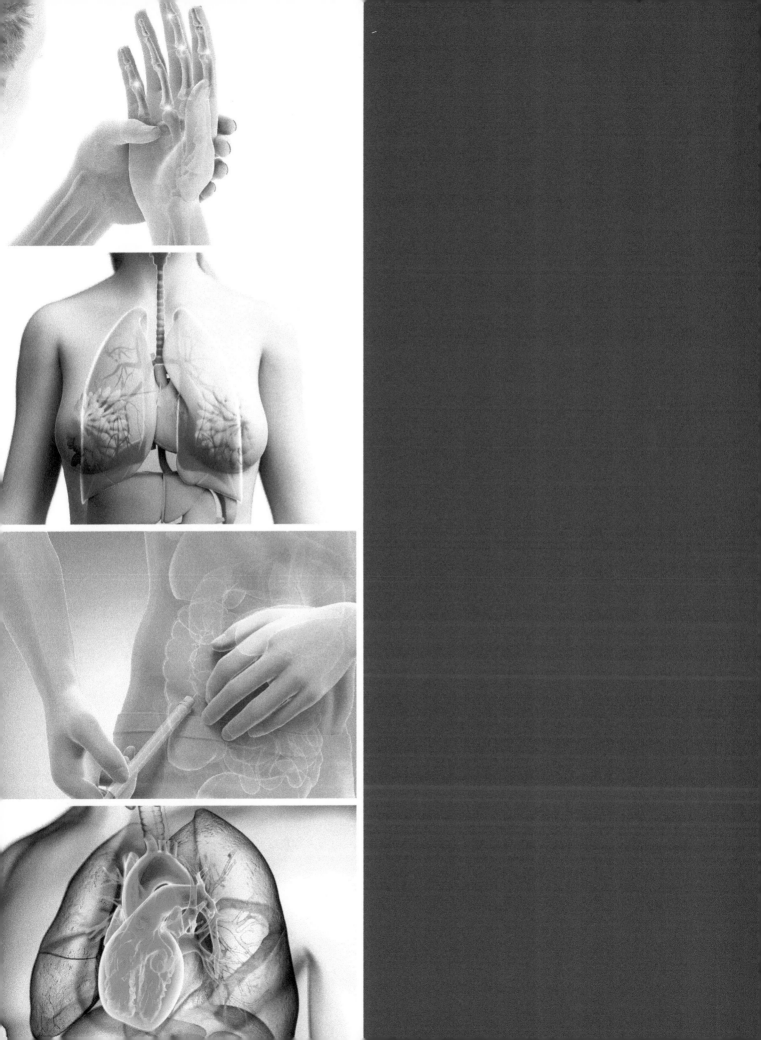

Diabetes mellitus type 2

34

Charlotte Gordon

Table 34.1 Modifiable and non-modifiable risk factors for T2D.

Non-modifiable risk factor for T2D	Modifiable risk factor for T2D
Genetics – history of T2D in a first degree relative	Excess body weight (obesity). BMI >35 kg/m² increases risk by 80-fold over 10 yr
Ethnicity – South Asian and Afro-Caribbean and may present at a younger age	Reduced physical activity – exercise increases insulin sensitivity and prevents obesity
Age – pancreatic beta cell function declines with age	High risk for T2D/pre diabetes
Previous gestational diabetes	Increasing waist circumference
	Steroid, HIV antiretroviral, antipsychotics medications

Table 34.2 HbA1c targets.

HbA1c level	Target (adults)
48 mmol/mol	Those managed with diet and lifestyle alone or in combination with a single drug not associated with inducing hypoglycaemia.
53 mmol/mol	Those managed with a drug associated with inducing hypoglycaemia.
>58 mmol/mol	People not adequately controlled by a single drug: • Reinforce diet, lifestyle, and treatment concordance. • Support the person to aim for HbA1c of 53 mmol/mol. • Intensify drug treatment.

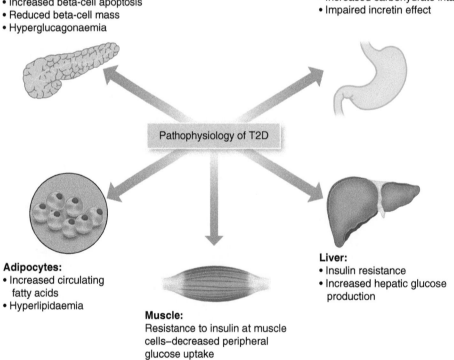

Figure 34.1 Pathophysiology of type 2 diabetes.

Pancreas:
• Decreased insulin secretion
• Increased beta-cell apoptosis
• Reduced beta-cell mass
• Hyperglucagonaemia

Stomach and gut:
• Increased carbohydrate intake
• Impaired incretin effect

Pathophysiology of T2D

Adipocytes:
• Increased circulating fatty acids
• Hyperlipidaemia

Muscle:
Resistance to insulin at muscle cells–decreased peripheral glucose uptake

Liver:
• Insulin resistance
• Increased hepatic glucose production

Long-term Conditions in Adults at a Glance, First Edition. Edited by Aby Mitchell, Barry Hill, and Ian Peate.
© 2023 John Wiley & Sons Ltd. Published 2023 by John Wiley & Sons Ltd.

Figure 34.2 HbA1c patient decision aid.

Aid to decision making when agreeing individualised HbA1c target – mark on the lines which statement is most applicable and depending on responses the best target can be decided

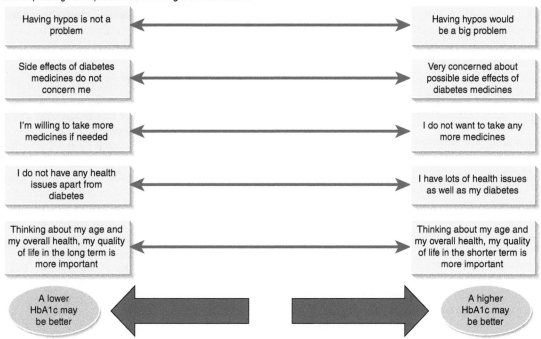

Table 34.3 Summary of medications for type 2 diabetes – refer to NICE (2022) for further detail.

Medication	Action	Place in treatment
Metformin (tablet)	• Reduces insulin resistance • Increases peripheral glucose uptake • Decreases hepatic glucose function • Only acts in presence of insulin	• First line treatment
SGLT2 – inhibitors (e.g.: dapaglaflozin – tablet)	• Block glucose reabsorption by the kidney • Cardioprotective	• First line in addition to metformin if established CVD or high risk • Alternative if metformin is not tolerated
Sulfonylureas (e.g.: gliclazide – tablet)	• Increases insulin production/secretion • Can cause hypoglycaemia	• Second line treatment
DPP4 (e.g.: sitagliptin – tablet)	• Inhibits DPP-4 activity, increasing post prandial active incretin (GLP-1, GIP) concentrations • Results in (glucose dependent) increased insulin and reduced glucagon secretion	• Second or third line treatment
Pioglitizone (rarely used – tablet)	• Increased tissue sensitivity to insulin	• Second or third line treatment
Insulin	• Stimulates glucose uptake by cells	• When dual therapy alone has not continued to control HbA1 to below the agreed threshold – use with or without other drugs
GLP-1 (e.g.: lixisenatide – injectable)	• Glucose dependent increased insulin and reduced glucagon secretion • Delays gastric emptying thereby reducing calorie intake through central appetite suppression – leads to weight loss	If triple therapy with metformin and two other oral drugs is not effective, not tolerated or contraindicated, consider triple therapy by switching one drug for a GLP-1 mimetic for adults with type 2 diabetes who: • have a body mass index (BMI) of 35 kg/m² or higher (adjust accordingly for people from Black, Asian and other minority ethnic groups) and specific psychological or other medical problems associated with obesity or • have a BMI lower than 35 kg/m² and: – for whom insulin therapy would have significant occupational implications or – weight loss would benefit other significant obesity related comorbidities.

Definition and epidemiology

Type 2 diabetes (T2D) is the most common form for diabetes mellitus accounting for over 90% of cases globally, however, many cases of T2D can be prevented or delayed with remission possible in some cases. T2D is a complex condition, affecting multiple organs, with an associated increased risk of micro and macrovascular disease; hyperglycaemia (elevated blood glucose) being the main clinical characteristic.

Since 1980, prevalence has doubled, currently affecting 8.5% of the global adult population; by 2025 global prevalence of T2D is set to increase particularly in low- and middle-income countries, demonstrating a persistently increasing global burden.

Previously considered a disease of middle age, T2D is observed in children, with risk factors similar to those in adults. A number of modifiable and non-modifiable risk factors contribute to the development of T2D (Table 34.1).

Altered pathophysiology

Two primary factors combine over time to cause T2D; a reduced secretion of insulin by pancreatic beta cells linked to reduced beta cell mass and additionally, reduced sensitivity/resistance to glucose at peripheral tissues (such as adipose, muscle, and the liver). It is unclear as to which is the primary defect. An imbalance between energy intake and expenditure then arises, this imbalance being responsible for disease progression in addition to environmental and genetic factors. Ongoing elevated blood glucose, over months and years, further impacts beta cell function and insulin secretion. Reduced sensitivity to insulin drives increased hepatic glucose production (gluconeogenesis), further compounding hyperglycaemia. Early intervention is essential to reduce disease burden and limit complications, of particular challenge given the patient may be asymptomatic. Often, there is a long pre-diagnostic period; globally, one third to one half of people with T2D may be undiagnosed. An overview of the pathogenesis of T2D is shown in Figure 34.1.

Diagnosis

Non-diabetic hyperglycaemia (NDH) or 'pre-diabetes' refers to the intermittent stage between normal glucose tolerance (function) and overt T2D; those in the pre-diabetes range are at increased risk of T2D and cardiovascular disease.

A two-stage risk assessment to prevent progression to T2D should be implemented, encompassing identifying those at high risk and as necessary, offering a blood test to confirm pre-diabetes or T2D.

The Leicester Risk Assessment Score is a validated seven question tool to identify those at high risk of pre-diabetes in UK multi-ethnic populations and considers the following components:
- Age
- Ethnicity
- Gender
- First degree family history of diabetes
- Antihypertensive treatment or history of hypertension
- Waist circumference
- BMI

Moderate risk for T2D refers to a high-risk assessment score where a blood test did not confirm that risk; high-risk refers to a fasting plasma glucose of 5.5–6.9 mmol/l or an HbA1c level of 42–47 mmol/mol, indicative of pre-diabetes.

Presenting features of T2D may include:
- Polydipsia (increased thirst)
- Polyuria (Increased urination)
- Blurred vision
- Unexplained weight loss
- Acanthosis nigricans (dark pigmentation of the skin suggesting insulin resistance)
- Presence of risk factors (see Table 34.1).

A diagnosis of T2D can be made in a symptomatic individual if HbA1c is 48 mmol/mol or above/fasting plasma glucose is 7.0 mmol/l or more/random plasma glucose of 11.1 mmol/l or more. If asymptomatic, repeat testing should be carried out, with the same testing method to confirm the diagnosis – if subsequent tests are normal, ongoing monitoring should be initiated as per clinical judgement. Practitioners should be aware of other additional features which may indicate other types of diabetes (for example rapid onset indicative of T1D).

Clinical management

Lifestyle interventions such as dietary modifications and moderate intensity exercise can reduce progression to T2D in those at high risk and are key to improved glycaemic control and associated reductions in complications for those with T2D. Structured education to address lifestyle modification is integral to diabetes care and should be offered at diagnosis with annual reinforcement. DESMOND is one such NICE approved validated programme which has demonstrated significant reductions in HbA1c and evaluates well with participants, improving their ability to self-manage. It is notable that attendance nationally is <10% but uptake can increase to 53% by training healthcare professionals to advocate the benefits of the programme.

HbA1c (see Chapter 32) targets for T2D (Table 34.2) should be individualised and agreed in consultation with the patient, taking lifestyle and pre-existing comorbidities into account (Figure 34.2). Targets should be relaxed in those who are frail if there is reduced likelihood of long-term benefit, if there are significant co-morbidities or if there is a high risk of hypoglycaemia and / or awareness is impaired. HbA1c should be measured initially every three months and then six-monthly once levels and blood glucose lowering therapies are stable. Self-monitoring of blood glucose by finger prick testing is not routinely required unless:
- using insulin
- evidence of hypoglycaemia
- risk of hypoglycaemia whilst driving/operating machinery
- the person is pregnant or planning pregnancy.

Drug therapies and regimens for T2D are complex, however, usual first line treatment is metformin, which works by decreasing gluconeogenesis from the liver and increases peripheral utilisation of glucose. SGLT2 inhibitors with proven cardiovascular benefit are now recommended as an additional first line treatment in those with established or at high risk of cardiovascular disease. Treatment escalation is required if agreed HbA1c targets are not met; ultimately, insulin may be required if dual therapy is not effective (Table 34.3).

Other clinical considerations – prevention and remission

The NHS diabetes prevention programme (DPP) is an evidence-based lifestyle change programme for adults at high risk of developing T2D to prevent of delay disease onset. The programme demonstrated significant reductions in weight and HbA1c, indicating that the DPP may lead to a reduction of T2D incidence.

In addition remission of T2D is also possible within six years of diagnosis through intensive weight management, achieved with significant reductions in calorie intake and weight loss (typically 15 kg or more). Whilst further evaluation of the approaches to prevention and management are needed, with focus on widening participation and addressing inequalities in uptake, approaches to care which are person-centred and encompass a holistic approach will contribute to limiting the burden of T2D.

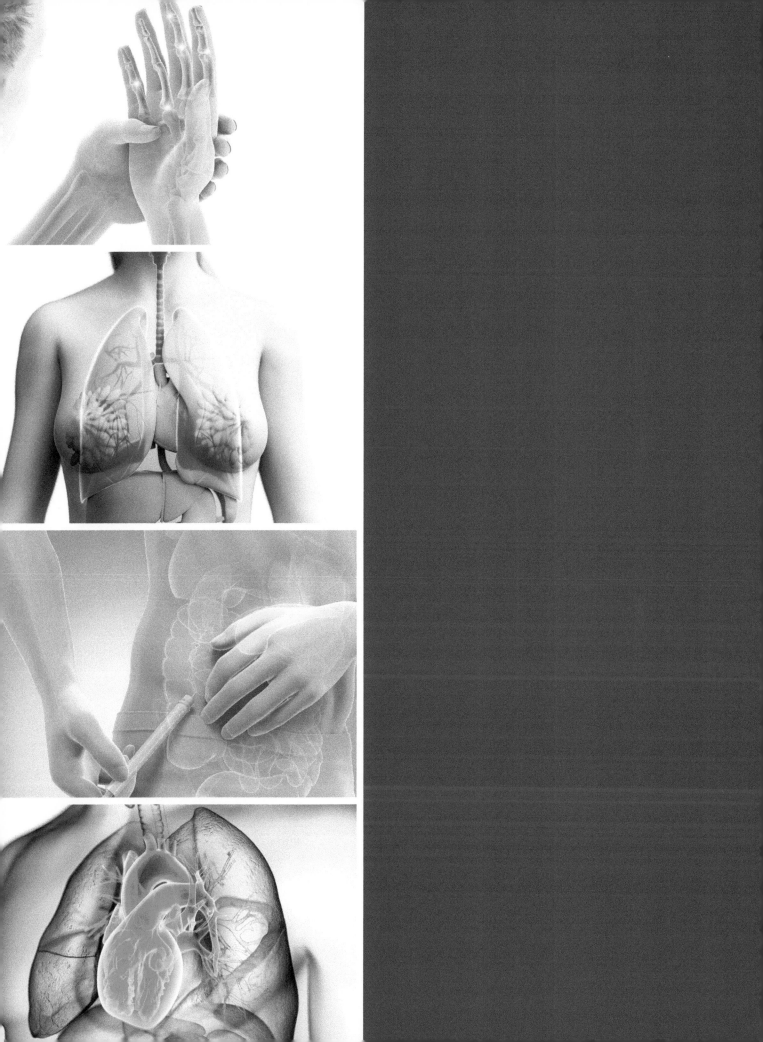

35 Dual diagnosis

Leticia Wedderburn and Daren Bailey

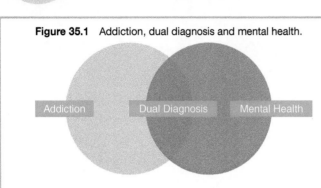

Figure 35.1 Addiction, dual diagnosis and mental health.

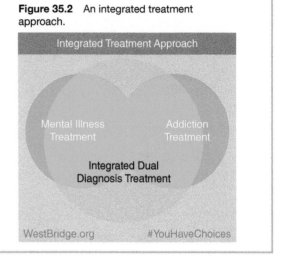

Figure 35.2 An integrated treatment approach.

Prevalence

In 2019, one out of every eight individuals, or 970 million people worldwide, experienced a mental condition, with anxiety and depression being the most frequent. Because of the COVID-19 pandemic, the number of people living with anxiety and depression disorders increased dramatically by 2020, such that over 95 million people with mental illnesses also have an alcohol or drug use condition, out of 460 million people with mental illnesses. This is due to a dual diagnosis.

A higher proportion of the population experience psychological discomfort than earlier estimates implied. In 2017, 271 million people, or 5.5% of the world population aged 15–64 years, were projected to have taken drugs in the preceding year. The most often used substance is cannabis. Dual diagnosis rates of 20–37% across all mental health settings and 6–15% in addiction settings have been observed. The number of people living with a mental health condition and who abuse drugs has risen by 62%, especially among those with schizophrenia.

Definition

The phrase 'dual diagnosis' is defined as 'a broad spectrum of mental health and drug use disorders that an individual may experience concurrently.' The link between these two conditions is complicated as substance use or misuse can aggravate or change the course of mental ill health; intoxication and/or substance dependency can cause psychological symptoms; and substance use and/or withdrawal can cause psychiatric symptoms or disorders.

A variety of alternative meanings can also be found in other sources; as a result, no precise definition has been adopted in the UK or elsewhere, leading in the development of exclusive policies. The harmful impact of drug or alcohol use on those who have mental health problems is referred to as dual diagnosis. People with dual diagnoses include those who use non-prescribed medications or alcohol to self-medicate in order to regulate their mental illness or those whose mental health deteriorates significantly as a result of using drugs or alcohol recreationally; or those who are at high risk of developing mental health issues as a result of major drug or alcohol use or addiction.

Both mental health and drug or alcohol treatment agencies recognise that dual diagnosis is a concern. It is estimated that 55–70% of persons who seek drug abuse therapy also have mental health issues, even if they have never sought mental health care. Figure 35.1 shows the relationship between addiction, dual diagnosis and mental health.

Symptoms

'Co-morbidity' refers to the presence of two or more conditions in the same person; dual diagnosis is also referred to as co-morbidity. With regards to a person's long-term addiction recovery strategy, it is critical to never disregard the indications of a mental health or behavioural condition. Recovering from substance misuse or drug addiction is not always easy, and the healing process can be challenging. Treatment providers recommend investigating signs and symptoms to determine whether a patient has a dual condition.

The symptoms of a dual diagnosis vary considerably across people, and symptoms will depend on the type of drug consumed as well as the degree of their co-occurring disorder.

Indications of dual diagnosis include rapid changes in general behaviour, such as changes in sleep patterns (insomnia or excessive sleep), or trouble managing daily tasks and obligations. Avoiding previously loved events or social activities, suggesting social disengagement from friends, relatives, and those who offer support, which is also a key indicator of service users experiencing a dual illness. Some indications include disillusioned thinking or cognitive problems, reluctance to seek or cooperate with therapy, suicidal thoughts or actions, financial concerns, poor performance at school or job, and aggressive, violent, or reckless conduct.

Treatment approach

The most successful treatment for dual diagnosis is an integrated strategy in which both mental health and substance abuse concerns are addressed concurrently and by the same treatment provider or team. Individual or group counselling, peer support, meditation, and lifestyle changes can all be used to treat mental illnesses (for instance, exercise, healthy eating, and quality sleep). Substance abuse treatment may include detoxification, management of withdrawal symptoms, counselling, and behavioural therapy. Figure 35.2 advocates and integrated treatment approach.

Substance abuse is a chronic relapsing disorder. It is critical that professionals have a realistic and long-term perspective on therapy, as various treatments may be required at different phases. For dual diagnosis programmes to successfully interact with service users who are typically non-concordant with mental health and drug abuse care, forceful outreach is required. A history of trauma can often render the onset of co-occurring disorders. There is frequently a lack of motivation for change, as well as a lack of awareness of the negative impact of their substance use on their mental health. As a result, prior to addressing substance abuse concerns, participation may entail addressing practical or other challenges.

It is necessary to have a relapse prevention programme, which helps people understand the triggers that lead to their drug abuse and explore building skills to deal with high-risk circumstances. This is an important part of relapse prevention as it allows people to have more control over their risky behaviours. Relapse prevention is integrated in individual care plans, and the programme provides guidance and assistance to mental health professionals.

The first step in treating a co-occurring condition is detoxification in a safe setting to eliminate narcotics from the person's system. From there, rehabilitation may begin in the form of counselling and programmes tailored to each unique patient. Behavioural modification treatments can aid in the treatment of both diseases by changing thought patterns and behaviours. Individual treatment approaches can be modified or adapted to better address two separate ailments rather than just one. The duration of the dual diagnostic team's interaction with the service user should not be limited. The programme focuses on the service user's requirements, and the length of engagement is determined by the individual's need and development.

36 Diverticular disease

Laura Park and Claire Ford

Table 36.1 Key terminology.

Diverticulum	This is a small pouch which protrudes out from the wall of the colon
Diverticula	The term used to describe more than one diverticulum
Diverticulitis	A condition when a single diverticulum or several diverticula become inflamed or infected
Diverticulosis	A condition where diverticula are present without symptoms

Figure 36.1 Large intestine. Source: Peate, I. Anatomy and Physiology for Nursing and Healthcare Students at a Glance (2e), 2022, p. 64, Figure 28.2.

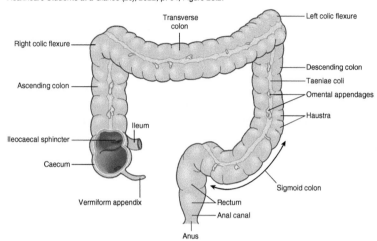

Table 36.2 Structures of the large intestine and associated functions.

Structure	Function
Ascending colon	The ascending colon, otherwise referred to as the right colon is the first section of the colon, extending from the caecum to the hepatic flexure. It averages 12–25 cm in length, 2.5 in. in diameter and is lined with smooth muscles that contract and move the contents along its length. Inside pouches increase the surface area, allowing for more absorption of the nutrients from the partially digested food passed on from the small intestine.
Transverse colon	This is the second part of the colon and as its name suggests, it traverses the abdomen, from the right colic flexure to the spleen. It is also the longest part of the colon and plays an important role in the absorption of water and salt.
Descending colon	This is the part of the colon, starting at the splenic flexure, which moves downwards towards the pelvis and is approximately 10–15 cm. It also plays a role in the absorption of nutrients but is mostly responsible for storing the remains of digested food, in the form of a stool, before they are eliminated.
Ileocaecal sphincter	This is a sphincter muscle, which assists with the passage of digested food materials from the small intestine into the large intestine. It is situated at the junction of the ileum and the colon.
Caecum	The caecum is a pouch-shaped part of the large intestine where digesting food enters after leaving the small intestine.
Sigmoid colon	This is located at the end of the large intestine, nearest the rectum and is an s-shaped loop, approximately 40 cm in length and can expand and contract depending upon the amount of faecal material being stored.
Haustra	These are small segmented pouches of the bowel, which are formed by folds, created by circumferential contraction of the inner muscular layer of the colon.
Anal canal	This is the last part of the gastrointestinal tract and is approximately 3–4 cm long. The function of the anal canal is the maintenance of faecal continence and defaecation, which is controlled by the anal sphincters and puborectalis muscle.

Introduction

Diverticular disease and diverticulitis (see Table 36.1) are related digestive conditions that affect the large intestine (colon) (see Figure 36.1 and Table 36.2). In diverticular disease, small pouches develop in the lining of the intestine (see Figure 36.2) and when bacteria and undigested food are left in a diverticulum pocket, they can become infected and inflamed and the condition develops into diverticulitis.

Although diverticular disease is a common condition of the large bowel, the exact causes of how these diverticula develop, remain uncertain. It is estimated that the condition affects 5–10% of the population aged over 45 years and is most common in western countries, with USA, Europe and Australia experiencing the highest prevalence of reported cases. Neither gender is more susceptible to diverticular disease and diverticulitis; however, it is reported that men are more likely than women to develop the condition at a younger age.

Risk factors

There are several environmental and non-environmental risk factors associated with the development of diverticular disease and diverticulitis.

Long-term Conditions in Adults at a Glance, First Edition. Edited by Aby Mitchell, Barry Hill, and Ian Peate.
© 2023 John Wiley & Sons Ltd. Published 2023 by John Wiley & Sons Ltd.

Figure 36.2 Diverticular pouch. Source: Peate, I. Medical-Surgical Nursing at a Glance – (Nursing and Healthcare), 2016, p. 64, Figure 30.1.

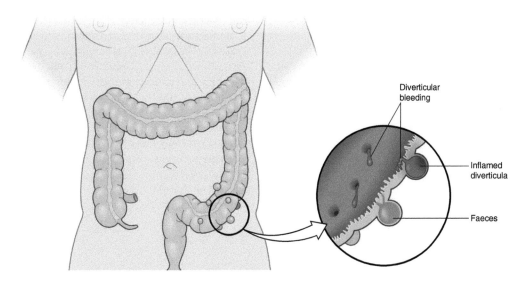

Table 36.3 Complications associated with diverticular disease.

Bleeding	Whilst bleeding is a common complication, experienced by approximately 15% of people with diverticular disease or diverticulitis, it is usually painless, and resolves quickly in 70–80% of cases.
Urinary problems	Diverticulitis can lead to inflamed and swollen sections of the bowel pressing on the bladder. This can cause pain upon urination and increased frequency.
Fistulae	These are abnormal tunnels that are formed between two previously unconnected parts of the body. These tunnels then have the potential to enable the transmission of bacteria, triggering infections.
Abscess	These form outside of the large intestine and are the most common complication of diverticular disease.
Peritonitis	This can occur when infected pouches in the colon rupture, leading to the spread of infection and microorganisms into the lining of the abdomen. This can be life-threatening.
Obstruction	Infections can lead to scarring and blockages within the large intestine and a total blockage is a medical emergency.

- **Age:** The walls of the large intestine become weakened with age and the pressure exerted by the hard stool as it passes through the weakened walls can cause diverticula to form.
- **Obesity:** Complications of the condition have also been found to be more prevalent in people with a high body max index (BMI). Current research suggesting that proinflammatory cytokines from visceral body fat could contribute to increased rates of chronic inflammation within the colon.
- **Diet:** A diet low in fibre is linked to the development of diverticular disease and diverticulitis. Fibre helps to soften stools and enable larger stools to form, which aids the speed at which the stool passes through the colon. This results in less pressure being exerted on the walls of the intestine, which may be weakened with age.
- **Dehydration:** Reduced or inadequate fluid intake leads to stools which lack moisture, and this results in greater pressure being exerted on the walls of the colon, as they try to move the stool towards the rectum. Additionally, a lack of fluid can cause a build-up of waste and bacteria, which can lead to inflammation and irritation.
- **Physical activity:** Lack of physical activity has been found to slow the passage of stools and increase pressure against the colon wall.
- **Genetics:** Individuals who have diverticular disease in their family, i.e. close relatives, are more likely to develop this condition.

- **Smoking:** Chemicals present in tobacco can damage and weaken the lining of the colon.
- **Medication:** individuals with diverticular disease should avoid non-steroidal anti-inflammatory drugs and opioid analgesia, as they may increase the risk of diverticular perforation.

Signs and symptoms

Signs and symptoms of diverticular disease and diverticulitis can vary between individuals and symptoms can overlap with other conditions, such as pancreatitis, bowel cancer, irritable bowel syndrome and colitis. It is therefore recommended that individuals seek support from their health-care provider if they experience a change in symptoms or develop any new symptoms, in order to determine if the symptoms are related to an existing or new condition.

Symptoms can start suddenly with the most common being described as lower abdominal pain, with intermittent cramps and pain often located in the left side of the abdomen, which increases when eating. While left-sided pain is common it is important to be aware that in a minority of people and individuals of Asian heritage, pain may be experienced in the right lower quadrant. Other signs and symptoms include changes in bowel habits such as diarrhoea and/or constipation, and mucus or blood in the stool (see Table 36.3). When the condition develops into diverticulitis, the pain may become more severe and constant, and individuals may also experience nausea and vomiting, develop a high temperature, and feel fatigued and generally unwell. Complications such as peritonitis and bowel obstruction can be life-threatening and must be treated as a medical emergency.

Treatment and management

There is no cure for diverticular disease; however, there are management and treatment strategies that can be used to minimise symptoms and reduce the risk of diverticulitis and further complications.

- **Diet:** Eating a high-fibre diet (30 g of fibre a day) may help ease the symptoms of diverticular disease. Fibre can be found in nuts, cereals and starchy foods, vegetables, beans and pulses, and fresh or dried fruits.
- **Hydration:** Oral intake should be increased along with fibre, as fibre acts like a sponge and soaks up fluid, making softer stools. This results in less pressure being exerted on the walls of the intestine, as the stools traverse the length of the colon. Increasing fibre and not fluid can lead to constipation.
- **Other lifestyle advice:** Increase exercise/activity, lose weight and reduce/stop smoking.
- **Medication:** There is no medication to cure/treat the general symptoms; however, paracetamol can be used to relieve pain, an antispasmodic can be prescribed if the person has abdominal cramping and antibiotics may be required if the condition has progressed to diverticulitis. Analgesics such as aspirin and ibuprofen, should be avoided as they can irritate the gastrointestinal tract and prescribed bulk-forming laxatives to ease constipation should be reviewed regularly as they can worsen the condition.
- **Surgery:** Serious complications of diverticulitis may require surgical intervention, and this usually involves removing the affected section of the colon. This is known as a colectomy, and it can be carried out via open or laparoscopic surgery.

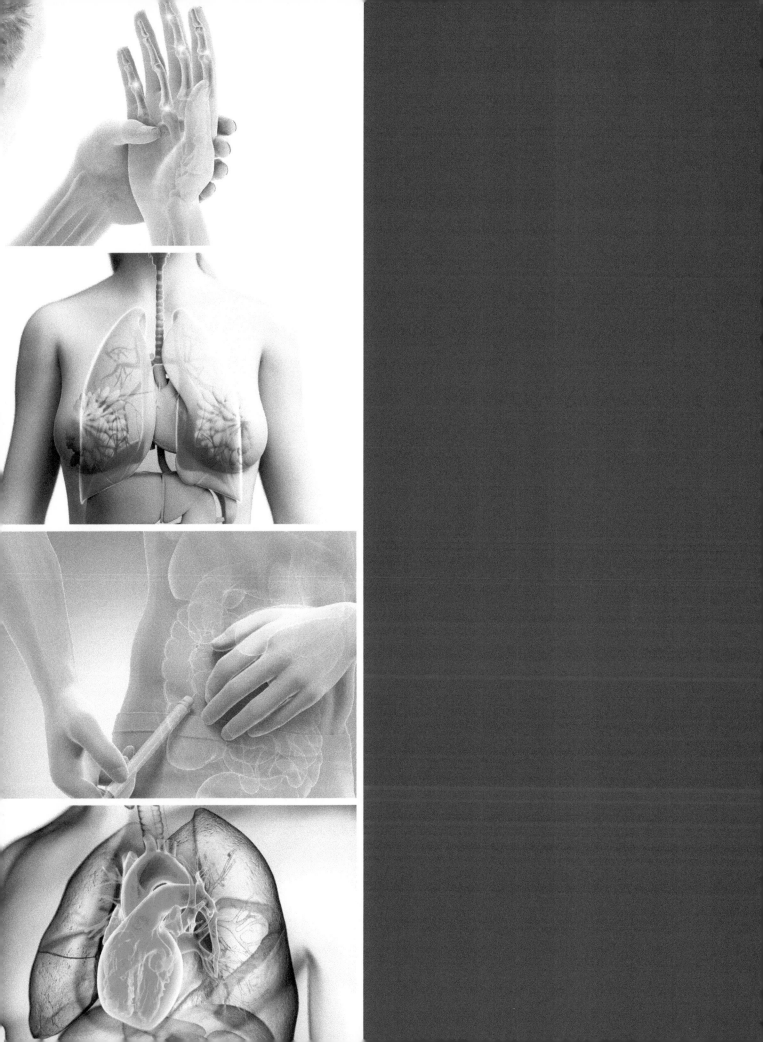

37 Epilepsy

Ian Peate

Source: WHO (2022).

Box 37.1   Epilepsy key facts

- Epilepsy is a chronic noncommunicable disease affecting people of all ages.
- Globally approximately 50 million people have epilepsy; it is one of the most common neurological diseases.
- Around 80% of people with epilepsy live in low- and middle-income countries.
- Up to 70% of people living with epilepsy could live seizure-free if properly diagnosed and treated.
- The risk of premature death in people with epilepsy is up to three times higher than it is for the general population.
- Three-quarters of people with epilepsy living in low-income countries do not receive the treatment they need.
- In many parts of the world, people living with epilepsy and their families experience stigma and discrimination.

Box 37.2   Features that could be part of an epilepsy syndrome

- Types of seizures
- Age at which the seizures begin
- Causes of seizures
- If the seizures are genetic
- Part of the brain affected
- Triggers provoking seizures
- Severity of seizures
- Frequent of seizures
- Seizure patterns

Figure 37.1   Signs and symptoms of a seizure.

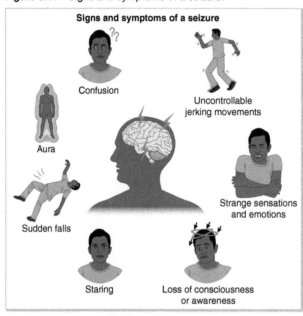

Table 37.1   Terminology used by the DVLA in relation to epilepsy.

Term	Meaning
Awake seizures	Seizures that start when the person is awake.
Asleep seizures	Seizures occurring as the person is falling asleep, whilst they are asleep or as they are waking up.
Anti-epilepsy drugs	Medication for epilepsy.
Group 1	Cars and motorbikes.
Group 2	Buses, coaches and lorries.
Permitted seizures	Types of seizures where the person can drive even if they are still having these seizures, after a pattern has been established over a given period of time.
Isolated seizures	First and single unprovoked seizure in a person who has not had any other unprovoked seizures during the past 5 years. This also includes more than one seizure if all of the seizures have occurred within a 24 h period.

Long-term Conditions in Adults at a Glance, First Edition. Edited by Aby Mitchell, Barry Hill, and Ian Peate.
© 2023 John Wiley & Sons Ltd. Published 2023 by John Wiley & Sons Ltd.

Epilepsy is a chronic non communicable condition. For some people it is long-term condition, a lifetime condition; for others they may have it for a period of their life and their epilepsy may dissipate. See Box 37.1.

Disability

Epilepsy can be classified as a disability. The Equality Act 2010 seeks to ensure that people are treated fairly and not discriminated against. This aspect of legislation applies to employment, school and learning, and accessing services including health and care services.

Epilepsy is deemed a disability when it greatly affects a person's ability to undertake everyday activities over a long period of time. Epilepsy may be described as a hidden disability as it is not usually obvious that a person has the condition unless they have a seizure. Those with epilepsy are protected by the Equality Act.

Epilepsy

Epilepsy is a neurological disorder whereby a person experiences frequent seizures. The International League Against Epilepsy has described epilepsy as a disease of the brain that is defined by any of the following conditions:

• At least two unprovoked seizures that occur more than 24 hours apart.
• One unprovoked seizure and a likelihood of further seizures similar to the general recurrence risk (at least 60%) after two unprovoked seizures, occurring over the next 10 years.
• Diagnosis of an epilepsy syndrome.

An epilepsy syndrome is defined as a group of signs and symptoms usually occurring together. The features of a syndrome can include, for example, the age the seizures began, gender, the types of seizures, the part of the brain affected (see Box 37.2).

Diagnosis of epilepsy is complex; it is made by a neurologist and a range of diagnostic investigations are undertaken. These include an electroencephalogram and an MRI scan. An in-depth assessment is undertaken and is based on finding out what happened before, during and after seizures. A neurological examination is performed and bloods are taken so as to illuminate differential diagnoses.

Treatment is based on findings; generally anti-epileptic drugs are prescribed. Most people with epilepsy can become seizure-free by taking one anti-epileptic drug. Others may be able to decrease the frequency and intensity of their seizures by taking a combination of medications. Determining the right medication and dosage can be complex. Individual assessment is needed and consideration give to the person's condition, frequency of their seizures, age and other factors when choosing which medication to prescribe. Usually a single medication is prescribed at a relatively low dose; the dose may be increased gradually until seizures are controlled.

Seizures

A seizure is the temporary occurrence of signs or symptoms due to atypical excessive or synchronous neuronal activity in the brain. Seizures can appear as a disturbance of consciousness, behaviour, cognition, emotion, motor function or sensation. An isolated seizure can be the result of toxins, metabolic, structural and infectious factors. These should not be mistaken with epilepsy.

Convulsive status epilepticus is a prolonged convulsive seizure that lasts for five minutes or longer or recurrent seizures occurring one after the other without any recovery in between.

Focal seizures

These originate in networks limited to one hemisphere of the brain and can be localised or more widely distributed. Focal seizures are divided into those where there is retained awareness or impaired awareness.

Generalised seizures

Originating in bilaterally distributed networks and can include cortical and subcortical structures of the brain (but not necessarily the whole cortex). Generalised seizures are divided into motor and non-motor (absence) seizures. See Figure 37.1 for some signs and symptoms of a seizure.

Care and support

People with epilepsy are entitled to free prescriptions for their anti-epileptic medication, as well as for any other prescribed drugs. Those on a low income or benefits, may be able to claim back some of the travel cost to some medical appointments. The cost of some equipment designed specifically to help people with disabilities, for example, a seizure alarm system does not include the tax payment.

A person may be entitled a health and care assessment depending on their epilepsy. The assessment is usually undertaken by an occupational therapist, taking place in the person's home and determines whether the individual has any physical or health problems, social or housing needs and what support they are already receiving be this from family or friends. When the assessment has been undertaken and it has identified that the person has needs which meet the local authority's criteria, then relevant community care services have to be provided. These may include meals, home help, adaptations to the home (for example, installing a shower or personal alarm) and access to leisure activities.

Driving and epilepsy

If a person has a driving licence, it is a legal requirement to tell the driving agency about any medical condition that could influence the person's ability to drive and this includes epilepsy. This is a condition of having a driving licence. If the person has a driving licence and has had a seizure of any kind, in most instances they must stop driving.

In the UK if a person has had a seizure they must inform the driving agency, for example, Driver and Vehicle Licencing Agency (DVLA) in Great Britain. They are required to inform their insurance company. How the driving regulations will apply will depend on the type of seizures the person is having, the type of seizures they have had previously and the type of licence the person has (Group 1 or Group 2). See Table 37.1 for some of the terminology used by the DVLA.

38 Heart failure

Barry Hill

Figure 38.1 Red flags for heart failure.

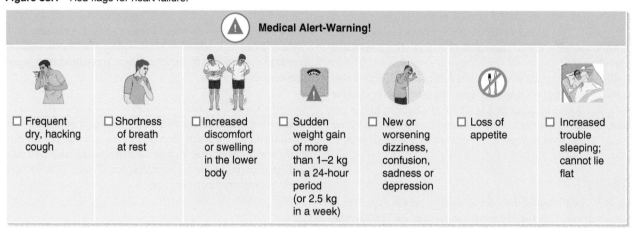

⚠ **Medical Alert-Warning!**

- ☐ Frequent dry, hacking cough
- ☐ Shortness of breath at rest
- ☐ Increased discomfort or swelling in the lower body
- ☐ Sudden weight gain of more than 1–2 kg in a 24-hour period (or 2.5 kg in a week)
- ☐ New or worsening dizziness, confusion, sadness or depression
- ☐ Loss of appetite
- ☐ Increased trouble sleeping; cannot lie flat

Table 38.1 Symptoms of heart failure.

Heart failure can be ongoing (chronic), or it may start suddenly (acute). Heart failure signs and symptoms may include:
- Shortness of breath with activity or when lying down
- Fatigue and weakness
- Swelling in the legs, ankles and feet
- Rapid or irregular heartbeat
- Reduced ability to exercise
- Persistent cough or wheezing with white or pink blood-tinged mucus
- Swelling of the belly area (abdomen)
- Very rapid weight gain from fluid accumulation
- Nausea and lack of appetite
- Difficulty concentrating or decreased alertness
- Chest pain if heart failure is caused by a heart attack

Table 38.2 Stages of heart failure.

Stages of heart failure are provided as a class. This ranges from 1 to 4, with 1 being the least severe and 4 being the most severe:
- Class 1 – No symptoms during normal physical activity
- Class 2 – Comfortable at rest, but normal physical activity triggers symptoms
- Class 3 – Comfortable at rest, but minor physical activity triggers symptoms
- Class 4 – Unable to carry out any physical activity without discomfort and may have symptoms even when resting

Long-term Conditions in Adults at a Glance, First Edition. Edited by Aby Mitchell, Barry Hill, and Ian Peate.
© 2023 John Wiley & Sons Ltd. Published 2023 by John Wiley & Sons Ltd.

The term heart failure makes it sound like the heart is no longer working at all and there is nothing that can be done. Heart failure means that the heart is not pumping effectively. Congestive heart failure is a type of heart failure that requires medical attention, although sometimes the two terms are used interchangeably. The body depends on the heart's pumping action to deliver oxygen- and nutrient-rich blood to the body's cells. When the cells are nourished properly, the body can function normally. With heart failure, the weakened heart cannot supply the cells with enough blood. This results in fatigue and shortness of breath and some people experience coughing. Everyday activities such as walking, climbing stairs or carrying groceries can become very difficult. Heart failure is a serious condition, and usually there is no cure. But many people with heart failure lead a full, enjoyable life when the condition is managed with heart failure medications and healthy lifestyle changes. It is also helpful for people with heart failure to have the support of clinical experts, family and friends who understand the condition.

Causes of heart failure

The most common causes of heart failure are myocardial infarction (MI) (heart attack) – which can cause long-term damage to the heart, affecting how well the heart can pump; hypertension (high blood pressure) – putting strain on the heart, which over time can lead to heart failure; and cardiomyopathy (diseased heart muscle). Heart failure can also be caused by heart valve disease; abnormal heart rhythms (arrhythmias); congenital heart conditions – heart problems from birth; endocarditis – a viral infection affecting the heart muscle; some cancer treatments, such as chemotherapy; excessive alcohol consumption; anaemia – a lack of oxygen carrying haemoglobin or red blood cells in the blood; and thyroid gland disease. Also, heart failure can be caused by pulmonary hypertension (raised blood pressure in the blood vessels that supply the lungs). This condition can damage the right side of the heart, leading to heart failure. In some cases, the pulmonary hypertension itself is caused by an existing heart condition. Amyloidosis is another cause and occurs when abnormal proteins, called amyloid, build up in organs (such as the heart, kidneys, and liver) and tissues. This affects how the organs work. If amyloidosis affects the heart, it is called cardiac amyloidosis – or 'stiff heart syndrome' – and can lead to heart failure. The red flags and symptoms of heart failure can be seen in Figure 38.1 and Table 38.1.

Diagnostic tests

There are four classes of heart failure (Table 38.2), and a range of tests that can be used for diagnostic purposes:

• Blood tests – to check whether there is anything in the blood that might indicate heart failure or another illness. Blood tests usually explore kidney and thyroid gland health and measure cholesterol levels. They also check for anaemia, which can occur with a reduction of healthy red blood cells.

• B-type natriuretic peptide (BNP) blood test. Brain natriuretic peptide is a substance the body makes. The heart releases it when heart failure develops. It is turned into N-terminal pro-brain natriuretic peptide (NT-proBNP). Levels of both can be higher in people with heart failure. These tests can be used to help clarify if a patient's shortness of breath is caused by heart failure.

• An electrocardiogram (ECG) – this records the electrical activity of the heart to check for problems with heart rate and rhythm. ECGs record the electrical impulses travelling through the heart muscle.

• An echocardiogram (echo) – a type of ultrasound scan where sound waves are used to examine the heart.

• Breathing tests include spirometry and a peak flow rate.

• A chest X-ray – to check whether the heart's bigger than it should be, whether there's fluid around the heart and inside the lungs (a sign of heart failure), or whether a lung condition could be causing the symptoms.

• Ejection fraction (EF). It is a measure of how much blood is pumped out of the heart each time it beats. A normal amount is between 55% and 75%, which means that over half of the blood volume is pumped out of the heart with each beat. Heart failure may happen because of a low EF.

• Cardiac catheterisation (coronary angiogram). This measures coronary artery disease (arterial blockages).

• Cardiac MRI utilises images to explore heart muscle or tissue damage surrounding the heart.

• CT coronary angiogram. It uses an X-ray and a contrast dye to observe for coronary artery disease.

• Myocardial biopsy. In this test, a small, flexible biopsy catheter is inserted into a vein in the neck or groin and takes a small piece of the heart muscle. This test can diagnose certain types of heart muscle diseases that cause heart failure.

• Stress test. The heart can become 'stressed' with exercise and can offer valuable data to support the decision making of clinicians.

Treatments

Treatment of heart failure depends on the underlying cause, and this will direct the main treatment to prevent further deterioration. Heart failure can be cured if it has a treatable cause. If the causes are due to coronary heart disease, then the patient may require coronary stents or bypass surgery. If there is a heart valve cause, then the defective valve will need surgery to repair or replace the valve. All heart failure patients will need lifestyle changes, including eating a healthy diet, exercising regularly, and stopping smoking and watching fluid intake and reduce alcohol consumption. They are also likely to need medication. Many people need to take three to four different types which have evidence to show they strengthen the heart and improve prognosis. This includes beta-blockers, ACE inhibitors, ARNI and SGLT2 inhibitors. Other medicines, such as diuretics, may be used to help with the symptoms. In cases where patients are seen to be experiencing continued deteriorating heart function despite the best and optimal medication, the following may be considered cardiac resynchronising therapy. In very severe heart failure conditions, a specialised type of pacemaker has shown to benefit and improve symptoms as well as prolonging life by resynchronising the contractility of the two main pumping chambers of the heart. Additionally, some patients maybe suitable for cardiac transplant. If there is no scope for recovery and the condition deteriorates then in suitable patients, a heart transplant may be considered. Treatment for heart failure usually aims to control the symptoms for as long as possible and slow down the progression of the condition. Treatment will usually be needed for life.

39 HIV

Ian Peate

Long-term Conditions in Adults at a Glance, First Edition. Edited by Aby Mitchell, Barry Hill, and Ian Peate.
© 2023 John Wiley & Sons Ltd. Published 2023 by John Wiley & Sons Ltd.

Figure 39.1 Treatment pathway. Source: NICE (2022).

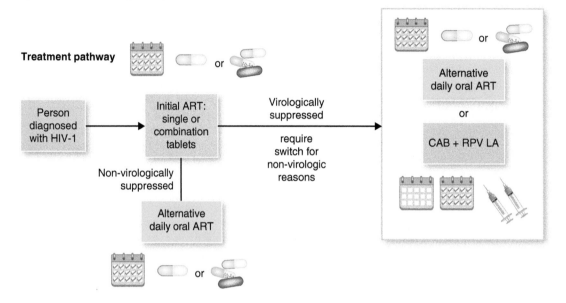

Box 39.1   HIV and AIDS

- HIV is a virus that damages the immune system, the body's normal defence against illness.
- If HIV is left untreated, then the individual's immune system becomes weaker and weaker until it is no longer able to combat life-threatening infections and diseases.
- With treatment, people who are living with HIV can experience a long and healthy life.
- AIDS is a set of symptoms and illnesses that develop at the final stage of HIV infection, if HIV is left untreated.
- Regularly testing for HIV means that antiretroviral treatment can be made available if required.

Source: Adapted from the British Medical Journal (2022).

Table 39.1 HIV medicines. Source: Tseng et al. (2015); British National Formulary/NICE (2022).

Treatment	Description
Nucleoside reverse transcriptase inhibitors (NRTIs)	Drugs that inhibit HIV replication by preventing the viral RNA being converted to DNA by the reverse transcriptase enzyme for insertion into the human genome, prevents HIV from being replicated.
Protease inhibitors (PIs)	PIs reduce viral load by competing with HIV proteins to bind with CD4 T-cell proteases. Prevents the viral proteins from binding and maturing for release in new viral particles.
Non-nucleoside reverse transcriptase inhibitors (NNRTIs)	NNRTIs target the same stage of HIV replication as NRTIs, binding to the reverse transcriptase produced by HIV, changing the properties of the enzyme's active site, reducing its activity and as such inhibiting HIV replication. Combining these mechanisms of action and specifically two NRTIs and a PI or NNRTI, in highly active antiretroviral therapy (HAART) regimens were more effective at reducing viral load to undetectable levels as opposed to using the treatments as monotherapies. HAART regimens are also known as combinatorial ART (cART).
Fusion Inhibitors (FIs)	Prevents the HIV virus envelope from fusing to the host CD4 T-cell membrane and thus, infection.
Co-receptor antagonists	Stabilises the CCR5 co-receptor on CD4 T cells in a configuration which HIV cannot bind to; this prevents infection.
Integrase strand transfer inhibitors (INSTIs)	INSTIs interact with the integrase enzyme produced by HIV particles, preventing it from inserting the viral DNA produced via reverse transcription into the genome of host CD4 T cells, preventing viral replication.
Attachment Inhibitors	A novel class of HIV ARTs bind to the gp120 protein on the outer surface of HIV, preventing HIV from binding to and entering CD4 T cells.

HIV as a long-term condition

Efforts to treat and eradicate human immunodeficiency virus (HIV) remain out of reach. Over 30 years after HIV-1 was identified, HIV remains an ongoing medical issue. HIV-1 was first isolated in 1983.Situating HIV as a long-term condition has not replaced the predominant image of HIV as a serious, communicable disease, a disease which is ultimately fatal. Living with HIV has changed. HIV has transformed from an acute illness with a poor prognosis to a long-term condition with a near normal lifespan and reduced health and social support. Those providing care and support to people with HIV have had to change in how they practice moving from supporting and managing people who are acutely unwell, applying their palliative and terminal care skills, to now developing skills in preventative health and health promotion related to healthy lifestyles.

HIV meets the definition of a long-term condition as it is a condition that cannot, at present be cured; however, it can be controlled by medication and other therapies. HIV is an illness as with other illnesses combining issues of ageing where management and support across primary, secondary and tertiary care services will be required. The presence of co-morbidities are associated with the natural ageing process, however in older people with HIV there is an increased risk of co-morbidities associated with the long-term use of antiretroviral therapy (ART), chronic inflammation linked with HIV and constant immune stimulation.

Human immunodeficiency virus

HIV is a retrovirus that is unable to self-replicate (see Figure 39.1). HIV infects and uses human CD4 T cells it replicates and spreads throughout the body. Over time, HIV particles destroy CD4 T cells, reducing a person's capacity to fight pathogens, leaving the person vulnerable to opportunistic infections. Those who develop several such infections are experiencing the most advanced stage of HIV and are diagnosed with acquired immune deficiency syndrome (AIDS). Whilst there is currently no cure for HIV/AIDS, treatments have been developed and the majority of people with HIV will never progress to developing AIDS, they are living with a long-term condition. See Box 39.1.

Treatments for HIV

In the UK, for the majority of people receiving treatment for HIV-1, this comes in the form of daily lifelong antiretroviral tablets. The aim of this treatment regimen is to keep the viral load at such a low level so that it cannot be detected or transmitted between people.

A major advance in highly active antiretroviral therapy (HAART) is the establishment of single-tablet fixed-dose combination products for nucleoside reverse transcriptase inhibitors (NRTI) and protease inhibitor (PI) backbone regimens, improving patient adherence. The two-drug cART regimens have reduced side-effects and toxicity and are a central part of changing treatment options. A wide range of treatments for HIV have been developed over the years since the first ART. There are seven distinct mechanisms of action for HIV medicines; see Table 39.1.

Long-acting therapy

Long-acting therapy has emerged as a treatment option introduced, in part, as a result of user need and people not wanting to think about living with HIV every day and taking medication daily. For some people living with HIV and having to remember to take tablets every day is a constant reminder of HIV. Having to take daily multi-tablet regimens can be difficult because of drug-related side-effects and toxicity as well as other psychosocial issues such as stigma or changes in lifestyle.

The first long-acting injection cART regimen for HIV has been approved in the UK (rilpivirine and cabotegravir) and will be available on the NHS for HIV-1 in adults: if the viral load is lower than 50 per millilitre of blood while taking a stable dose of antiretrovirals and if the person has tried non-nucleoside reverse transcriptase inhibitors or integrase inhibitors in the past, their condition has not become resistant to these and their viral load has stayed low while taking them. The treatment is to be administered as two separate injections every two months, after an initial oral lead-in period. These are important treatment options for those who already have good levels of concordance to daily tablets and who may wish to opt for an injectable regimen requiring less frequent dosing. Long-acting therapies have the potential to make a big difference to the health and well-being of people living with HIV, liberating people from the daily reminder of their long-term condition. Further developments in the field may mean that new products will become available with different mechanisms of action, for example, the introduction of ultra-long-acting regimens, requiring dosing perhaps twice yearly.

Stigma and HIV

Stigma remains an issue for those living with HIV having a negative impact on an individual's health and relationships. Stigma impacts every area of life; internalised or self-stigma are significant obstacles to those with HIV living satisfied and happy lives. Those with HIV still face discrimination and prejudice from friends, family, employers or when trying to access services or facilities. Sharing HIV status is not a one-off act, it is ongoing throughout the individual's life, requiring the person to be resilient and confident with their diagnosis, characteristics that not all people with HIV can keep up all of the time.

Supporting those with HIV

Those living with HIV should have equitable access to services that encourage self-management of HIV including the offer of support and provision of information about HIV, treatment options, healthy living with HIV, diet and lifestyle and enhancing health and well-being and access to rehabilitation services. People with long-term conditions are central to any processes that will enhance their health and well-being, supported by health and social care professionals as they express their own needs and make their own decisions on their own priorities occurring through a process of information-sharing, shared decision-making and action planning.

Despite phenomenal scientific advances, HIV is still incurable; the virus can however, be controlled by innovative treatment regimens where people are required to take their treatment for life. Health and care providers are best placed to monitor long-term health issues and to support people living with HIV who wish to manage their own care.

Hypertension

Barry Hill

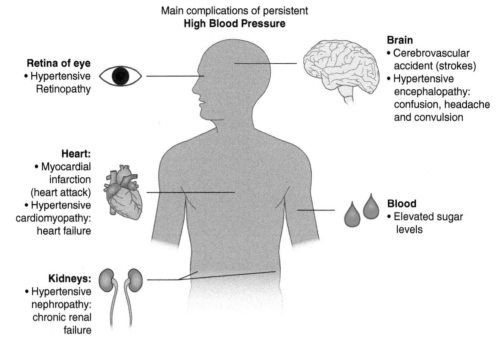

Figure 40.1 Complications of hypertension.

Main complications of persistent
High Blood Pressure

Retina of eye
• Hypertensive Retinopathy

Brain
• Cerebrovascular accident (strokes)
• Hypertensive encephalopathy: confusion, headache and convulsion

Heart:
• Myocardial infarction (heart attack)
• Hypertensive cardiomyopathy: heart failure

Blood
• Elevated sugar levels

Kidneys:
• Hypertensive nephropathy: chronic renal failure

Table 40.1 Symptoms of high blood pressure.

High blood pressure rarely has noticeable symptoms. The following can be symptoms of high blood pressure:
• Blurred vision
• Nosebleeds
• Shortness of breath
• Chest pain
• Dizziness
• Headaches
More than one in four adults in the UK have high blood pressure, but many will not know they have it. Many people with high blood pressure feel fine. Healthy adults over 40 are recommended to have their BP checked at least once every five years. However, if they are at increased risk of high blood pressure, they should have it checked more often, ideally once a year.

Long-term Conditions in Adults at a Glance, First Edition. Edited by Aby Mitchell, Barry Hill, and Ian Peate.
© 2023 John Wiley & Sons Ltd. Published 2023 by John Wiley & Sons Ltd.

Blood pressure is the force exerted by circulating blood against the walls of the body's arteries, the major blood vessels in the body. Hypertension is when blood pressure is too high. Blood pressure is written as two numbers. The first (systolic) number represents the pressure in blood vessels when the heart contracts or beats. The second (diastolic) number represents the pressure in the vessels when the heart rests between beats. They're both measured in millimetres of mercury (mmHg). The NHS (2022) identifies high blood pressure being 140/90 mmHg or higher (or 150/90 mmHg or higher over the age of 80); ideal blood pressure is usually considered to be between 90/60 mmHg and 120/80 mmHg. The blood pressure equation is Blood Pressure (BP) = Cardiac Output (CO) × Peripheral Vascular Resistance (PVR) (BP = CO × PVR).

Causes

There isn't always an explanation for the cause of high blood pressure, but most people develop high blood pressure because of their diet, lifestyle, or medical condition. Sometimes high blood pressure runs in families and can also worsen with age. People living in deprived areas are at higher risk of having high blood pressure, and it is also more common if a person is of black African or black Caribbean descent. Even in these cases, people can improve blood pressure by changing to healthy diets and being active.

The following factors can all increase the risk of having high blood pressure:
- drinking too much alcohol
- smoking
- being overweight
- not doing enough exercise
- eating too much salt.

In a very small number of people, the cause of high blood pressure can be identified. This is sometimes referred to as secondary hypertension. For example, an abnormal production of hormones from the adrenal glands can lead to high blood pressure. If medication is prescribed to treat such a hormonal condition, then blood pressure should return to normal. Other causes of secondary hypertension include kidney disease, diabetes, and some medicines, such as oral contraceptives and some over the counter and herbal medicines.

Pathophysiology

Hypertension is a chronic elevation of blood pressure that, in the long-term, causes end-organ damage and results in increased morbidity and mortality. Blood pressure is the product of cardiac output and systemic vascular resistance. Patients with arterial hypertension may have an increase in cardiac output, an increase in systemic vascular resistance, or both. In the younger age group, the cardiac output is often elevated, while in older patients increased systemic vascular resistance and increased stiffness of the vasculature play a dominant role. Vascular tone may be elevated because of increased α-adrenoceptor stimulation or increased release of peptides such as angiotensin or endothelins. The final pathway is an increase in cytosolic calcium in vascular smooth muscle causing vasoconstriction. Several growth factors, including angiotensin and endothelins, cause an increase in vascular smooth muscle mass termed vascular remodelling. Both an increase in systemic vascular resistance and an increase in vascular stiffness augment the load imposed on the left ventricle; this induces left ventricular hypertrophy and left ventricular diastolic dysfunction. The autonomic nervous system plays an important role in the control of blood pressure. In hypertensive patients, both increased release of, and enhanced peripheral sensitivity to, norepinephrine can be found. In addition, there is increased responsiveness to stressful stimuli. Another feature of arterial hypertension is a resetting of the baroreflexes and decreased baroreceptor sensitivity. The renin–angiotensin system is involved at least in some forms of hypertension (e.g., renovascular hypertension) and is suppressed in the presence of primary hyperaldosteronism. Elderly or black patients tend to have low-renin hypertension. Others have high-renin hypertension, and these are more likely to develop myocardial infarction and other cardiovascular complications.

Complications

Among other complications, hypertension can cause serious damage to the heart. Excessive pressure can harden arteries, decreasing the flow of blood and oxygen to the heart. This elevated pressure and reduced blood flow can cause chest pain, also called angina; and heart attack, which occurs when the blood supply to the heart is blocked, and heart muscle cells die from lack of oxygen. The longer the blood flow is blocked, the greater the damage to the heart. Heart failure occurs when the heart cannot pump enough blood and oxygen to other vital body organs. Irregular heartbeat can lead to a sudden death. Hypertension can also burst or block arteries that supply blood and oxygen to the brain, causing a stroke. In addition, hypertension can cause kidney damage, leading to kidney failure. See Figure 40.1.

Recommendation for practice

The World Health Organization (WHO) is supporting countries to reduce hypertension as a public health problem. In 2021, the WHO released a new guideline on the pharmacological treatment of hypertension in adults. The publication provides evidence-based recommendations for the initiation of treatment of hypertension. It gives recommended intervals for follow-up, and describes controlling blood pressure with targeted control. There are several medicines used to treat high blood pressure including ACE inhibitors, angiotensin receptor blockers (ARBs), calcium-channel blockers, diuretics, alpha-blockers (doxazocin), and beta-blockers. Most people need to take more than one type of medicine to lower their blood pressure; however taking two or more medicines often has greater effect. See Table 40.1.

Inflammatory bowel disease

41

Claire Ford and Laura Park

Figure 41.1 Common types of inflammatory bowel disease.

Inflammatory bowel disease (IBD)

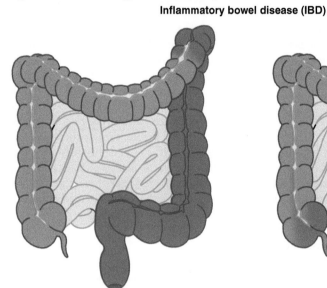
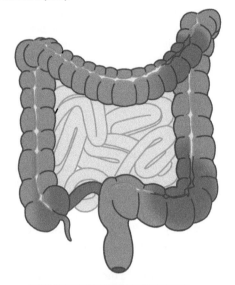

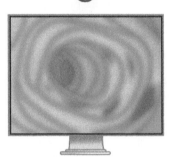
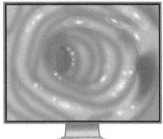

Ulcerative colitis

Crohn's disease

Table 41.1 Diagnostic procedures for IBD.

Blood tests	Platelets, red and white blood cells, and C-reactive protein (CRP) are examined for inflammation markers.
Stool tests	Examined for levels of calprotectin, a protein biomarker that the body releases when there is inflammation.
Ultrasound/ CT/ MRI	Used to build a 3D image of the body to help locate areas of inflammation.
Endoscopic procedures	Endoscopies, including sigmoidoscopy, colonoscopy, and gastroscopy enable detailed visual examination of the inside of the digestive tract. This is carried out with the use of a small camera mounted to the end of a lighted tube.
Biopsy	These are usually taken during an endoscopic procedure. The specimens are sent to the laboratory and examined under a microscope to check for inflammation.

Long-term Conditions in Adults at a Glance, First Edition. Edited by Aby Mitchell, Barry Hill, and Ian Peate.
© 2023 John Wiley & Sons Ltd. Published 2023 by John Wiley & Sons Ltd.

Inflammatory bowel disease (IBD) is used as an umbrella term to describe conditions that cause chronic inflammation (including periods of relapse and remission) of the gastrointestinal (GI) tract, the two most common of which are Crohn's disease and ulcerative colitis. IBD can often be confused with irritable bowel syndrome (IBS); however, whilst these are both gastrointestinal disorders and have similar symptoms, there are differences between the two conditions. IBS is a syndrome that is classified as a functional gastrointestinal disorder, caused by interactions between the brain and gut, whereas IBD is categorised as an immune-mediated inflammatory disease that has the potential to permanently harm the intestines and increase individual's risk of developing colon cancer. IBD is a lifelong disease, with increasing global prevalence. In the UK there are over 300 000 individuals living with IBD and in the USA this number is thought to be around 3.1 million.

The causes of IBD
While the exact cause of IBD remains unanswered, several factors have been found to contribute to the risk of IBD development:
- genetics
- environmental risk factors (i.e. virus, medication, smoking)
- imbalance or changes in the intestinal bacteria
- abnormal immune system response.

Crohn's disease
Although it is mostly reported to affect the ileum in the small intestine, Crohn's can affect any part of the GI tract. The submucosa becomes inflamed and this usually occurs in patches known as 'skip lesions' which give a cobblestone appearance. Crohn's also has the potential to affect other areas of the body, causing inflammation in the eyes, joints and skin. See Figure 41.1.

Ulcerative colitis
Ulcerative colitis differs from Crohn's as the disorder results in chronic inflammation of the large intestine and often the rectum and sigmoid colon. The ulcers that develop in ulcerative colitis start in the rectum's mucosa layer where they then spread to the large intestine. See Figure 41.1.

Signs, symptoms and investigations
Crohn's and ulcerative colitis have similar signs and symptoms. The most common symptoms associated with IBD are identified below (this is not an extensive list):
- **Abdominal pain:** Described as a cramping pain which can vary from mild to serve depending on the severity of the relapse.
- **Frequent diarrhoea and faecal urgency:** Urgency to open the bowels can be experienced, as well as episodes of diarrhoea, sometimes occurring up to 10–20 times a day.
- **Bleeding and/or mucus:** Blood and mucus can sometimes be seen in the stool and more bleeding can occur if further ulcers develop.
- **Anaemia:** Due to blood loss from the ulcers, individuals may become anaemic, which can lead to feelings of fatigue.
- **Weight loss:** This is seen more often in individuals with Crohn's as absorption of nutrients, protein and carbohydrates in the small intestine is impacted by the disease.

- **Mouth ulcers:** These are only related to Crohn's disease and not ulcerative colitis.
- Other common symptoms can include dehydration, constipation, pyrexia, loss of appetite, nausea, and vomiting.

IBD can also be diagnosed at any age using a range of tests and investigations (see Table 41.1); however, it is mostly identified before the age of 30.

Clinical management and interventions
While there is no cure for IBD, there are a number of effective treatments to help manage symptoms. However, as IBD is described as a condition that is associated with periods of relapse (flare-ups) and remission, individuals are continuously transitioning from periods of having no symptoms, to periods of managing mild to severe symptoms. For this reason, management of the symptoms can often be problematic and complex.
- **Medication:** such as steroids, immunosuppressants, analgesics and antispasmodics, can be used to reduce inflammation and manage symptoms such as pain. The medication will vary between individuals and the severity of the relapse and symptoms experienced.
- **Surgery:** This is often considered if medication is not effective, and the individual's quality of life is negatively impacted by the repeated periods of relapse. Examples of surgery include subtotal colectomy with ileostomy and colectomy with ileorectal anastomosis.
- **Diet:** A restricted or liquid diet can help, as it provides the gut with the opportunity to rest and heal; however, nutrition must be maintained therefore this should only be carried out under guidance and supervision from a health-care provider. It can also be beneficial for individuals who suffer from IBD to create a food diary, as some individuals find specific foods, such as spicy foods, that can trigger and/or help relieve symptoms. If absorption has been affected due to the inflammation caused by IBD, individuals may be advised to eat more of certain foods or advised to take vitamin supplements.
- **Supporting mental health:** Living with an IBD condition can trigger several emotions such as feelings of stress, fear, anxiety, and anger. Almost half of the people with Crohn's stated that their condition had affected their mental health. Referrals to specialised services may therefore be required to support their overall health and well-being.

Complications of IBD
There are several complications associated with IBD the most common of which include:
- **Fistulas:** Around one in three people with Crohn's develop a fistula, a tunnel that connects an organ to another part of the body. In Crohn's, these tunnels often can connect the bowel to another internal organ, such as the vagina, bladder, or skin.
- **Narrowing of the gut:** While rare in individuals with ulcerative colitis, ongoing inflammation can result in narrowing, known as a stricture, which can make it difficult for the passage of stools. In Crohn's, it is the repeated cycle of inflammation and healing that cause scar tissue to form causing strictures.
- **Toxic mega colon:** This complication is seen more in individuals with ulcerative colitis especially when the inflammation is extensive and severe, resulting in the bowel wall thinning and the colon becoming bloated with gas.
- **Perforation:** This is rare but can occur if a blockage is caused by inflammation or stricture.

Multiple sclerosis

42

Barry Hill

Table 42.1 Types of MS.

1. Relapsing remitting MS

- Between 8 and 9 of every 10 people with MS are diagnosed with the relapsing remitting type.
- Someone with relapsing remitting MS will have episodes of new or worsening symptoms, known as relapses.
- These typically worsen over a few days, last for days to weeks to months, then slowly improve over a similar time period.
- Relapses often occur without warning but are sometimes associated with a period of illness or stress.
- The symptoms of a relapse may disappear altogether, with or without treatment, although some symptoms often persist, with repeated attacks happening over several years.
- Periods between attacks are known as periods of remission. These can last for years at a time.
- After many years (usually decades), many, but not all, people with relapsing remitting MS go on to develop secondary progressive MS.
- In this type of MS, symptoms gradually worsen over time without obvious attacks. Some people continue to have infrequent relapses during this stage.
- About two-thirds of people with relapsing remitting MS will develop secondary progressive MS.

2. Primary progressive MS

- Between 1 and 2 in every 10 people with the condition start their MS with a gradual worsening of symptoms.
- In primary progressive MS, symptoms gradually worsen and accumulate over several years, and there are no periods of remission, though people often have periods where their condition appears to stabilise.

Figure 42.1 Progressive course of multiple sclerosis. https://onlinelibrary.wiley.com/doi/full/10.1111/joim.13045.

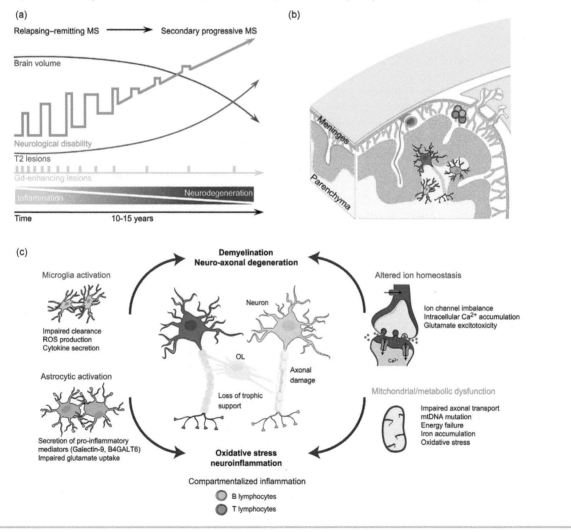

Multiple sclerosis (MS) is an autoimmune disease that can affect the brain and spinal cord, causing a wide range of potential symptoms, including problems with vision, arm or leg movement, sensation, or balance. It's a lifelong condition that can sometimes cause serious disability, although it can occasionally be mild. In many cases, it's possible to treat symptoms. Average life expectancy is slightly reduced for people with MS. It's most diagnosed in people in their 20s, 30s, and 40s although it can develop at any age. It is 2–3 times more common in women than men. MS is one of the most common causes of disability in younger adults. There are two types of MS including relapsing remitting MS: and primary progressive MS (Table 42.1).

Incidence and prevalence

It is estimated that there are over 130 000 people with MS in the UK, and that nearly 7000 people are newly diagnosed each year This means that around one in every 500 people in the UK has MS, and that each week, 130 people are diagnosed with MS. The cause of MS is unknown. It is believed that an abnormal immune response to environmental triggers in people who are genetically predisposed results in immune-mediated acute, and then chronic, inflammation. The initial phase of inflammation is followed by a phase of progressive degeneration of the affected cells in the nervous system. MS is a potentially highly disabling disorder with considerable personal, social and economic consequences. People with MS live for many years after diagnosis with significant impact on their ability to work, as well as an adverse and often highly debilitating effect on their quality of life and that of their families. MS is an autoimmune disorder that affects those with a genetic susceptibility to environmental risk factors. Active inflammation is the best-understood component of the disease and is associated with demyelination, the neurodegenerative phase of disease, whereas grey-matter pathology and compartmental inflammation described in the meninges over time are more enigmatic and self-perpetuating. Recent pathological and imaging findings have also revealed that inflammation arises at any stage of MS.

Pathophysiology

MS refers to the plaques that form in the CNS combined with inflammation, demyelination, axonal injury, and axonal loss. These plaques are found in the brain and spinal cord, essentially in the white matter around the ventricles, optic nerves and tracts, corpus callosum, cerebellar peduncles, long tracts and subpial region of the spinal cord and brainstem, but also in the grey matter. During the early stages of the relapsing remitting course, the pathology is marked by important demyelination and a variable degree of axonal loss and reactive gliosis. Patients in general, present with focal inflammatory plaques that contain demyelinated axons, reduced number of oligodendrocytes, astrocyte proliferation with subsequent gliosis, transected axons, and perivenular as well as parenchymal infiltrates of lymphocytes and macrophages. In the progressive course, MS is dominated by diffuse grey and white matter atrophy and characterised by low-grade inflammation and microglial activation at the plaque borders combined with diffuse injury of the normal-appearing white matter outside the plaque. Inflammation, microglial activation, axonal and myelin injury occurring during this course are followed by secondary demyelination. In general, the patterns of tissue injured in patients presented with primary or secondary progressive course of MS are homogeneous. Typically, MS is regarded as a T cell-mediated autoimmune disorder with a predominance of CD8+ cells compared with other T-cell subsets, B cells or plasma cells. It is believed that this disease begins in inflammatory-induced lesions consisting mainly of CD8+ T cells, and CD4+ T cells, and activate microglia/macrophages. See Figure 42.1.

Treatments

Disease modifying therapies (DMTs) aren't a cure for MS, but they can reduce how many relapses someone has and how serious they are. They can also slow down the damage caused by relapsing multiple sclerosis that builds up over time. DMTs are treatments that could change (for the better) how your MS develops over time. DMTs are also known as 'disease modifying drugs' (DMDs) which are available as pills, injections, or infusions. A DMT could also be a treatment that uses stem cells. A DMT isn't a cure, but it could make a real difference to people with MS. The main benefits of taking one of the DMDs are fewer relapses, less severe relapses, and a reduction in the build-up of disability which can occur if people don't recover completely from relapses. DMDs work with different parts of the immune system to reduce the inflammation caused by MS to nerve cells in the brain and spinal cord. This helps reduce the number and severity of relapses.

43 Parkinson's disease

Kelley Storey and Annette Hand

Table 43.1 Cardinal features of Parkinson's.

Symptom	Definition
Bradykinesia	Bradykinesia means slowness of movement and is one of the cardinal manifestations of Parkinson's. Physical movements are much slower than normal, making everyday movements difficult. For example, walking can become a slow shuffle with very small steps.
Rigidity	Rigidity or stiffness is not experienced by every patient, it can be uncomfortable and very painful and contribute to a reduced range on motions it is sometimes called cogwheeling/lead pipe. Rigidity can prevent muscles form stretching, resulting in stopped posture, reduced facial expression.
Tremor	Tremor usually begins in the hand or the arm, it can sometimes be described as 'pill rolling' and is more likely to occur when the limb is relaxed or resting.

Table 43.2 The non-motor symptoms of Parkinson's.

Problem	Symptoms
Autonomic dysfunction	Urinary urgency and frequency Sexual dysfunction Hypotension Constipation Increased sweating
Sleep problems	Insomnia Rapid eye movement Restless legs syndrome Vivid dreams Nocturia
Neuropsychiatry problems	Depression Apathy Anxiety Dementia Confusion Delirium Panic attacks Obsessive behaviour
Sensory problems	Hyposmia Pain Paraesthesia
Other symptoms	Fatigue Diplopia Blurred vision Seborrhoea Weight loss Weight gain

Table 43.3 Medications used to treat Parkinson's.

Medication	Examples and mode of action
Dopamine precursor	• Levodopa (co-careldopa or co-beneldopa) is broken down in the brain to release dopamine. • Efficacy reduces with time, requiring larger/more frequent dosing. • Given with dopa-decarboxylase inhibitor (carbidopa/benserezide) to help prevent peripheral degradation of levodopa. • Available in standard release, dispersible preparation or prolonged release.
Dopamine agonists	• Examples include: rotigotine patch, ropinirole, pramipexole. • Ropinirole and pramipexole come in both standard and modified release. Pramipexole can come in either base or salt doses. • Directly activates post-synaptic dopamine receptors.
Monoamine oxidase B inhibitors	• Examples include rasagiline, selegiline, safinamide. • Often taken as adjunct (add on) therapy. • Inhibits the breakdown of dopamine, causing longer lasting effect.
Catechol-0-methyltransferase inhibitors	• Examples include entacapone, opicapone. • Can only be given as adjunct therapy. • Prevents the peripheral metabolism of levodopa.

Table 43.4 Medications to avoid in people with Parkinson's.

Symptom	Medications to avoid
Nausea and vomiting	Metoclopramide and prochlorperazine.
Agitation	Haloperidol, chlorpromazine, risperidone, olanzapine, chlorpromazine and fluphenazine.

Long-term Conditions in Adults at a Glance, First Edition. Edited by Aby Mitchell, Barry Hill, and Ian Peate.
© 2023 John Wiley & Sons Ltd. Published 2023 by John Wiley & Sons Ltd.

Parkinson's is one of the fastest growing neurological conditions in the world, for which there is no cure. Currently, it is estimated that there are over 145 000 people with Parkinson's in the UK, due to population growth and ageing this number is expected to rise to 172 000 by 2030. One in 37 people will be diagnosed with Parkinson's in their lifetime (Parkinson's UK 2018). Parkinson's is generally associated with older age but the age of onset for nearly 25% of individuals is younger than 65 years, and 5–10% being younger than 50 years at diagnosis.

Altered pathophysiology

Parkinson's is a complex neurodegenerative disorder that is characterised by the gradual depletion of dopamine in the brain. Dopamine is the chemical messenger that transmit signals from one nerve cell to another in the brain to co-ordinate activity. Motor symptoms of Parkinson's usually appear when at least 50–60% of dopamine levels have been lost. For most cases the underlying cause for developing Parkinson's remains unknown. There are genetic causes of Parkinson's in 3–5% of all cases. More men than women develop Parkinson's and as, yet we don't fully understand why, but is likely due to a combination of biological factors (hormones or genetics) and lifestyle factors (exposure to chemicals). Increasing age, repeated head injury, along with a number of lifestyle and environment factors have been identified as all increasing your risk of developing Parkinson's. However, exercise, smoking, drinking coffee and the use of anti-inflammatory drugs have been shown to reduce your risk of developing Parkinson's (Dorsey et al. 2020).

Parkinson's symptoms

For some people there are clues that they are developing Parkinson's; these are called prodromal non-motor features that predate the start of the motor features. These can include changes to smell and taste, constipation and acting out dreams during the rapid eye movement (REM) phase of sleep.

Motor symptoms usually start on one side of the body, then progress gradually over time (usually years) and can affect the whole body. There are many manifestations of Parkinson's, but the cardinal features of Parkinson's include bradykinesia (slowness and poverty of movement), rigidity (stiffness) and rest tremor (shaking) (see Table 43.1). Along with the motor features of Parkinson's, individuals can also develop a vast array of non-motor symptoms including autonomic dysfunction, sleep disorders, neuropsychiatric symptoms and gastrointestinal symptoms (see Table 43.2). People with Parkinson's often find that non-motor symptoms have a greater impact on their quality of life. As Parkinson's progresses the signs and symptoms worsen. People with Parkinson's can have increasing problems with poorer mobility, frequent falls, dysarthria (problems with speech), dysphagia (problems with swallowing), hallucinations and some individuals will also develop Parkinson's dementia. Symptoms can be life-changing and lead to marked disability.

Diagnosis of Parkinson's

The early identification and diagnosis of Parkinson's is important to ensure that individuals get the correct management and support. An individual will usually first present to their general practitioner (GP), and if they complain of symptoms of tremor, stiffness or slowness, Parkinson's should be suspected. The National Institute of Health and Care Excellence (NICE) guidance (2017) state that people with any of these symptoms, should be referred quickly, and untreated, to a specialist with expertise in Parkinson's. Parkinson's remains a clinical diagnosis; currently there are no tests or scans that can be performed to confirm the diagnosis. A diagnosis will be based on an individual's symptoms, medical, social and drug history and physical examination. Blood tests and brain scans may be ordered to exclude tumours or other brain pathology. An individual's motor and non-motor signs and symptoms will be assessed following the Movement Disorders Society Parkinson's diagnostic criteria. It is important that a specialist with expertise in Parkinson's is involved in the diagnostic stage as there are a number of different conditions, that appear similar to Parkinson's, but have different aetiology, treatment options and prognosis. Parkinsonism is the umbrella term for these conditions that causes slowness, stiffness or tremor and can include:

- Vascular Parkinsonism.
- Drug-induced Parkinsonism.
- Multiple system atrophy.
- Progressive supranuclear palsy.
- Corticobasal degeneration.
- Lewy body dementia.
- Normal pressure hydrocephalus.

The diagnosis of Parkinson's needs to be reviewed regularly, every 6–12 months, and reconsidered if atypical features develop or if individuals do not respond to Parkinson's treatment (NICE 2017). For individuals this may mean that it may take several months, or even years, to have a diagnosis of Parkinson's confirmed.

Clinical management

There are many ways that health-care professionals can encourage people with Parkinson's to contribute to their own health and well-being. Regular exercise has proven to be very beneficial to improve walking and balance. Advice on appropriate diet will also help to ease symptoms such as constipation, weight changes and reduced bone density.

At present there are no medical treatments that can slow, reverse or cure Parkinson's. Parkinson's medications (Table 43.3) can improve motor symptoms and work by increasing the dopaminergic activity in one of three main ways:

1 By directly replacing dopamine via a dopamine precursor.
2 By mimicking the effects of dopamine at the dopamine receptor sites.
3 Preventing the breakdown of dopamine by enzymes.

NICE Guidance for Parkinson's disease (NG71) provides treatment recommendations, depending on an individual's symptoms, and the severity of symptoms. Ultimately, the decision on when to start Parkinson's medication, and which one to commence, should be made on an individual basis, and in partnership with a specialist. There are a number of medications used to treat nausea, vomiting and agitation that should be avoided as these medications can make Parkinson's symptoms much worse (see Table 43.4).

Recommendations for practice

Parkinson's care needs to be person-centred and holistic. Motor symptoms can be controlled with Parkinson's medications and lifestyle changes. The non-motor symptoms can be tricky to control and need to be treated separately with a variety of pharmacological and non-pharmacological strategies. People with Parkinson's should be supported by a Parkinson's Specialist Nurse and a Movement Disease Specialist to provide ongoing information, support and advice. A multidisciplinary team approach is also vital to promote quality of life for people with Parkinson's.

Peripheral arterial disease

44

Aby Mitchell

Figure 44.1 Leg ulcer management. Source: Moffatt et al. (2007), Figure 5.1.

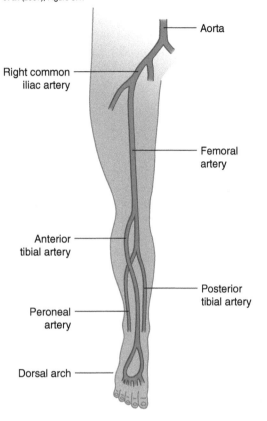

- Aorta
- Right common iliac artery
- Femoral artery
- Anterior tibial artery
- Posterior tibial artery
- Peroneal artery
- Dorsal arch

Table 44.1 Risk factors for PAD.

Family history	A family history of cardiovascular, cerebrovascular, or peripheral arterial disease and leg ulceration can be a predisposing factor of PAD.
Medical history	Diabetes mellitus is associated with early and rapid progression of atherosclerosis and a major risk factor of PAD. Hypertension accelerates the progression of atherosclerosis. It is not acknowledged to be a significant risk factor on its own but more significant in the presence of other risk factors. High serum cholesterol levels lead to an enhanced plaque formation. Raised levels of low-density lipoproteins increase the risk of atheroma. High-density lipoproteins protect against plaque formation. Other arterial diseases such as angina, myocardial infection, cardiac bypass/angioplasty, transient ischaemic attack, stroke and kidney disease all present as risk factors for PAD.
Smoking	Smoking is the most significant risk factor for PAD. Smoking damages the vascular endothelium and increases progression rate of atherosclerosis.
Exercise	Regular exercise of at least 150 minutes of moderate activity is thought to increase HDL levels (high-density lipoprotein or 'good' cholesterol) and protect against atherosclerosis.
Stress	Biological and immune responses associated with stress may predispose patients to atherosclerosis.
Age	Increase age is a risk factor of PAD.
Gender	The incidence of atherosclerosis appears to be higher in men under 70 but similar for both genders over 70. Oestrogen has a protective effect reducing LDL cholesterol.

Table 44.2 Interpretation of ABPI results (NICE 2021).

Less than. 0.5	Severe arterial disease.
Greater than 0.5 less than 0.8	Presence of arterial disease or mixed arterial/venous disease.
Between 0.8 and 1.3	Suggests no evidence of significant arterial disease.
Greater than 1.3	Suggests presence of arterial calcification commonly in patients with diabetes, rheumatoid arthritis, systemic vasculitis, atherosclerotic disease, and advanced chronic renal disease.

In the human body there are several different kinds of blood vessels. Arteries and arterioles are the vessels that transport oxygenated blood around the body away from the heart. Capillaries are tiny blood vessels that link the arterial and venous system by forming a delicate network of vessels close to body tissues. Blood vessels dilate, constrict, and pulsate to deliver blood which begins and ends at the heart.

Arteries

The arteries have two primary functions. They act as a network transporting oxygenated blood from the left ventricle of the heart to tissues. The second function is to sustain an adequate blood pressure and blood flow during the diastole. Other functions include cardiovascular haemostasis.

Arteries can be divided into three main groups:
- Elastic arteries – thick walls found near the heart, e.g. aorta.
- Muscular arteries – smooth muscle capable of greater vasoconstriction and vasodilation. Distribute blood to specific organs and parts of the body.
- Arterioles – determine the amount of blood flowing into organs and tissues.

The endothelium lines all the vessels and makes up the main part of the capillary wall. The role of the endothelium is significant in maintaining arterial pressure. It manages this by producing and releasing factors (i.e. nitric oxide) that have a relaxing effect on the

Long-term Conditions in Adults at a Glance, First Edition. Edited by Aby Mitchell, Barry Hill, and Ian Peate.
© 2023 John Wiley & Sons Ltd. Published 2023 by John Wiley & Sons Ltd.

smooth muscle of the artery which results in vasodilation, and endothelins which has a constrictive effect. In a healthy arterial network, the highly elastic walls and normal endothelial function ensures the sufficient flow of blood round the body.

The main arteries in the leg are depicted in Figure 44.1. These include the femoral artery, deep femoral artery, popliteal artery, posterior tibial artery, and anterior tibial artery. These arteries are responsible for providing a rich supply oxygenated blood and nutrients to the lower limb.

Peripheral arterial disease

It is estimated that approximately one in five people over 60 in the UK suffer from peripheral arterial disease (PAD). PAD is the failure of arteries to deliver sufficient blood to a particular part of the body which results in oxygen starvation (tissue ischaemia) and cellular death. When this occurs in the legs it is known as PAD. Over a prolonged period, this will lead to poorly nourished skin that is vulnerable to infection, has a reduced ability to repair and arterial leg ulcers. Risk factors for PAD are identified in Table 44.1.

Atherosclerosis

Atherosclerosis is a common cause of arterial disease which involves the formation of fatty plaques in the interior wall of the arteries. This causes the narrowing of the lumen (stenosis), hardening of the artery and endothelial dysfunction due to lipid accumulation. This occurs mainly in the larger and medium-sized vessels for example the aorta, its branches and the coronary arteries. These complications reduce pressure and the volume of blood reaching the arteries. This can also lead to heart disease and stroke. Symptoms are experienced when the lumen is occluded by 75%. Atherosclerosis effects different parts of the body in different ways.

Acute arterial thrombus or embolism

A thrombus is an unstable atheromatous plaque which can originate from an area of diseased artery and can result in thrombus formation for example atrial fibrillation. When the thrombus becomes mobilised it gets lodged in a smaller artery causing occlusion. Fat and air can also embolise. Assessments of patients suspected of should include the five P's:

- Pain
- Pallor
- Paraesthesia (burning or prickling sensation)
- Pulseless
- Perishing cold.

Inflammatory vascular disease

This is a rare, progressive, degenerative disease that affects the small and medium-sized arteries and veins. The artery wall becomes inflamed due to an occlusion that is surrounded by non-specific immune cells which deprive healthy cells local to the occlusion of oxygen and nutrients. This results in tissue ischaemia and symptoms such as intermittent claudication – fatigue, cramping, numbness, pain, tingling and weakness in a muscle group.

This is aggravated by exercise and relieved by rest. Chronic ischaemia results in persistent ischaemic rest pain.

Skin changes in PAD

- Limb colour may vary from pale to a mottled blue due to a lack of oxygen in the blood.
- Some limbs have a deep red/purple hue (dependant rubor). This is a result of the arteries in the foot vasodilating in an attempt to oxygenate the lower limb adequately which results in pooling of the arterial blood. This can give the appearance of cellulitis or a well-perfused limb. The colour remains the same regardless of being elevated or dependant.
- Dependant oedema.
- Diminished or absence of pedal pulses or monophasic sounds.
- Loss of sensation including numbness and tingling.
- Loss of hair – this is an indication perfusion is poor.
- Muscle weakness/wasting to the calf or thigh.
- Atrophic shiny skin.
- Arterial leg ulcer – these tend to be on the lower aspect of the limb at the foot or ankle. Have a punched-out appearance and can either be shallow or very deep exposing underlying structure. Granulation tissue (if present is pale), slough or necrosis is often present.

Assessment

Arteriogram

An invasive procedure used to visualise the inside/lumen of the blood vessels to check for blocked or damaged arteries.

Ankle brachial pressure index (ABPI)

ABPI assessment is a non-invasive way of assessing patient's vascular status and establishing if there is a presence of PAD by comparing systolic blood pressure at the ankle with the arm. A cuff is placed around each arm and ankle consecutively. ABPI testing is can also be referred as Doppler testing. The Doppler ultrasound is the traditional way of conducting an ABPI assessment. A Doppler machine uses high frequency waves to measure the amount of blood flowing through the patient's veins and arteries. ABPI assessment can be used as a more accurate identification of people at potential risk of arterial disease including amputation, heart attack and stroke. Table 44.2 interprets ABPI results.

Treatment

PAD is asymptomatic in patients with an ABPI >4.0. The goal of therapy with PAD is to control symptoms and improve quality of life. If PAD is diagnosed patient education is essential. Any lifestyle modifications can positively affect outcomes and optimise any surgical interventions. Patient lifestyle advice should include nutrition and dietary advice, understanding cholesterol control, exercise, and smoking cessation.

Patients with chronic ischaemia have an ABPI of less than 0.4 and ankle pressure of less than 50 mmHg. These patients are usually dependant on opiate analgesia. To manage these symptoms, it is important to encourage exercise to improve symptoms for 30 minutes at a time up to three times a week.

PAD is a common condition which can have a significant impact on patients' quality of life. Early assessment and intervention are important alongside patient education and lifestyle changes which can positively affect outcomes and optimise treatment and interventions.

45 Psoriasis

Ian Peate

Figure 45.1 Common locations of psoriasis. Source: Medical-Surgical Nursing at A Glance, 2016, chapter 41, p. 86, Figure 41.2. Wiley-Blackwell.

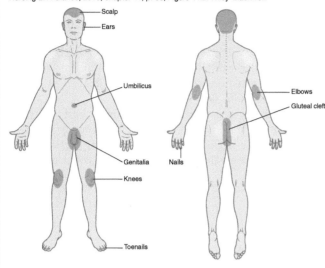

- Scalp
- Ears
- Umbilicus
- Genitalia
- Knees
- Toenails
- Elbows
- Gluteal cleft
- Nails

Figure 45.2 Types of psoriasis.

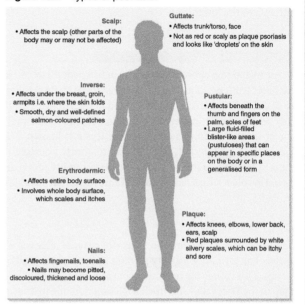

Scalp:
- Affects the scalp (other parts of the body may or may not be affected)

Guttate:
- Affects trunk/torso, face
- Not as red or scaly as plaque psoriasis and looks like 'droplets' on the skin

Inverse:
- Affects under the breast, groin, armpits i.e. where the skin folds
- Smooth, dry and well-defined salmon-coloured patches

Pustular:
- Affects beneath the thumb and fingers on the palm, soles of feet
- Large fluid-filled blister-like areas (pustuloses) that can appear in specific places on the body or in a generalised form

Erythrodermic:
- Affects entire body surface
- Involves whole body surface, which scales and itches

Nails:
- Affects fingernails, toenails
- Nails may become pitted, discoloured, thickened and loose

Plaque:
- Affects knees, elbows, lower back, ears, scalp
- Red plaques surrounded by white silvery scales, which can be itchy and sore

Figure 45.3 Normal skin and psoriasis.

Normal skin

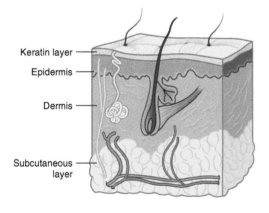

- Keratin layer
- Epidermis
- Dermis
- Subcutaneous layer

Psoriasis

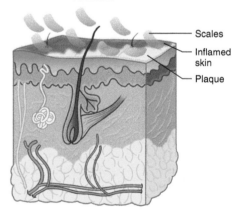

- Scales
- Inflamed skin
- Plaque

Box 45.1 A range of topical therapies available to manage psoriasis

- Emollients aim to lubricate the skin and ease scaling, as well as providing patient comfort.
- Coal tar ointments. These preparations have an antipruritic and anti-inflammatory effect (they may stain clothing).
- Dithranol is used to suppress cell proliferation.
- Vitamin D analogues such as calcipotriol, tacalcitol and calcitriol; used, amongst other things, to inhibit cell proliferation. Phototherapy can inhibit cell division in some forms of psoriasis.
- Retinoids, influence the activity of the epidermis.
- Topical steroids are used only for a short period.

Source: Adapted from Stephens (2021).

Long-term Conditions in Adults at a Glance, First Edition. Edited by Aby Mitchell, Barry Hill, and Ian Peate.
© 2023 John Wiley & Sons Ltd. Published 2023 by John Wiley & Sons Ltd.

Skin: long-term conditions

Chronic skin conditions can affect the young and old and can endure over the course of a lifetime. Many skin diseases themselves represent long-term conditions, for example, psoriasis, eczema, acne, vitiligo, leg ulcers and chronic sun damage that causes multiple skin cancers. People with long-term conditions related to other organs or systems, such as diabetes, HIV, transplants patients and cancer commonly get skin disease. There are some skin long-term conditions that are associated with increased physical and psychological disease, acne scarring, for example, is permanent. Acne results in long-term disabilities as well as difficulties in relationships and employment prospects.

Skin disease is one of the most common reasons for a new consultation in the primary care setting, it contributes immensely to long-term conditions with millions of people having dermatological long-term disorders such as eczema, psoriasis, acne, vitiligo as well as occupational skin disease. A number of other primarily non-dermatological long-term conditions generate considerable dermatological needs that are due to the disease itself or to its treatment with drugs and their consequences and side-effects. There are some dermatological long-term conditions, particularly psoriasis that are associated with substantial co-morbidity; metabolic syndrome and arthritis.

Psoriasis

Psoriasis is a chronic disease in which the immune system becomes overactive; this causes skin cells to multiply too rapidly, it has a relapsing–remitting course. Patches of skin become scaly and inflamed, most often on the scalp, back, elbows, or knees, but other parts of the body can be affected as well (see Figure 45.1). The aetiology of psoriasis is not fully understood, however what is known is that it involves a mix of genetic and environmental factors.

There are several forms of psoriasis (see Figure 45.2), this a non-infectious, inflammatory disorder that can appear as purple patches with grey scales on black skin. The patches can also appear as a dark brown colour. Generally, psoriasis patches appear more purple or brown on darker skin. However, for black people with lighter skin, these patches may look like those that appear on white skin: red, raised demarcation of skin patches with silvery whitish scales. The condition can vary from mild to severe. The patient may also experience an itch. If itching occurs, this causes the scales to shed easily. Psoriasis has the potential to cause the patient to feel ashamed and dirty.

From a pathophysiological perspective the cells of the basal layers of the epidermis reproduce and the more rapid upward progression of these cells through the epidermis causes incomplete maturation of the upper layer, there is an overproduction of skin cells (see Figure 45.3). Sometimes psoriasis is associated with arthritis, called psoriatic arthropathy. The rash associated with psoriasis can occur when the patient is experiencing an episode of arthritis. There is often a familial history associated with this condition.

Diagnosis is made on clinical presentation. Skin biopsy, skin swab, throat swab and blood tests as well as clinical examination are required to confirm diagnosis. There are a range of treatment options and this will include psychological support for the patient and the family. See Box 45.1 for a discussion of topical therapies to manage psoriasis. The health and care professional has a role to play in motivating and encouraging the patient to apply the therapies, adhering to the treatment regimen. It must be noted that whatever treatment is chosen is not a cure for the condition and no single treatment will suit everyone. It is essential that individual assessment is undertaken.

Living with psoriasis

Each person will experience psoriasis differently. For some the condition may not have a significant impact on their day-to-day life, however for other people the impact can be significant. For those who find that their day-to-day lives are affected, there are many things that can be disrupted by psoriasis, from work to relationships, getting a good night's sleep to wearing what the person wants to wear.

Work and employment

Changes at work may need to be made in order for people to effectively manage their condition at work. There may be certain occupations that could cause problems for people with psoriasis; these are very few. The Equality Act (2010) defines a 'disability' as a physical or mental impairment that has a substantial and long-term adverse effect on the ability to perform normal day-to-day activities. Psoriatic arthritis is treated as a continuing disability if it is likely to recur; employers are required to make reasonable adjustments to enable disabled employees to do their job. This could include providing equipment to help the employee operate technology or machinery, making changes to work premises so the employee has easy access, or permitting flexible working hours to accommodate medical appointments.

Triggers for psoriasis

There are a number of common triggers for an exacerbation of psoriasis; these can be different for different people. The trigger can be difficult to determine, many people never work out what their trigger is. Some triggers can include:

- **Infection.** Streptococcal infection (usually throat) is known to trigger guttate psoriasis.
- **Injury to skin.** The appearance of psoriasis around an injury is known as Koebner's phenomenon; this usually occurs around a wound, or a surgical scar, for instance.
- **Stress.** Can trigger psoriasis, making existing psoriasis worse.
- **Medications.** Medications can aggravate psoriasis that already exists or trigger an occurrence for the first time. One of the most significant is certain antimalarial drugs, such as chloroquine.
- **Diet.** Currently evidence regarding diet is inconclusive. However, some people believe that certain foods make their psoriasis worse or better.
- **Hormones.** The first appearance of psoriasis, for some people, occurs around the time of puberty or around the menopause. Psoriasis improves for many women whilst pregnant, although a small number find that the opposite occurs. Fluctuating hormone levels may have an effect on psoriasis in some people; there is no strong evidence-based to support this.
- **Alcohol and smoking.** Drinking alcohol might affect psoriasis as it is dehydrating and as such could dry skin out even more. It is unsafe to drink alcohol whilst using certain medications for psoriasis (methotrexate and acitretin). Smokers are more likely to develop psoriasis than non-smokers.

Pruritis

Pruritis can be one of the most constant and frustrating symptoms of psoriasis. Often the skin is itches as it is dry, keeping the skin well moisturised is important. Water and soap dry out the skin, moisturising after a bath or shower is recommended. Irritants such as soaps, bubble bath, detergents and any fabrics that seem to irritate should be avoided.

46 Rheumatoid arthritis

Jane Douglas and Karl Nicholl

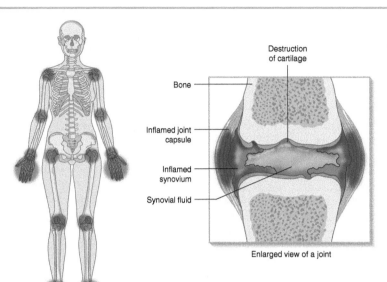

Figure 46.1 Joint pain and the destruction of cartilage. Source: Peate, I. Medical-Surgical Nursing at a Glance – (Nursing and Healthcare), 2016, chapter 41, p. 86, figure 41.2.

Destruction of cartilage

Bone

Inflamed joint capsule

Inflamed synovium

Synovial fluid

Enlarged view of a joint

Joint pain occurring in various joints

Table 46.1 Medication and Monitoring of RA.

Conventional synthetic disease modifying anti-rheumatic drugs (csDMARDs)	Frequency of administration and dosage	Blood monitoring frequency
Methotrexate (oral and sub-cutaneous [S/C])	Weekly – 5 to 25 mg	Every 2 weeks for 6 weeks, then monthly for 3 months, then every 3 months if stable
Leflunomide	Daily – 10 to 20 mg	As above
Sulfasalazine	Twice daily – titrate from 500 mg to 1 g twice daily	As above
Hydroxychloroquine	Daily – 200 to 400 mg	No monitoring required
Biologic drugs	**Frequency of administration and dosage**	**Blood monitoring frequency**
Abatacept	125 mg weekly sub-cutaneous (S/C) or every 4 weeks intra-venous (I.V.) infusion – by weight	At each infusion or every 3 months for S/C
Adalimumab	40 mg fortnightly S/C	Every 3 months
Certolizumab	400 mg every 2 wk S/C for 6 wk, then 200 mg every 2 wk thereafter	Every 3 months
Etanercept	25 mg twice weekly or 50 mg weekly	Every 3 months
Golimumab	50–100 mg monthly (depending on weight)	Every 3 months
Infliximab	I.V. at week 0, 2, and 6, then every 8 weeks	At each infusion
Rituximab	I.V. Infusion 1 g at week 0 and week 2 then every 6 months	At each infusion
Tocilizumab	I.V. Infusion every 4 weeks at 8 mg/kg or weekly S/C 162 mg	At each infusion or every 3 months for S/C
Targeted synthetic janus kinase inhibitor drugs (JAKs)	**Frequency of administration and dosage**	**Blood monitoring frequency**
Baricitinib	Daily – 2 to 4 mg depending on age and eGFR	Every 3 months
Filgotinib	Daily – 100 to 200 mg depending on age and eGFR	Every 3 months
Tofacitinib	5 mg twice daily	Every 3 months
Upadacitinib	Daily – 15 to 30 mg depending on age and eGFR	Every 3 months

Long-term Conditions in Adults at a Glance, First Edition. Edited by Aby Mitchell, Barry Hill, and Ian Peate.
© 2023 John Wiley & Sons Ltd. Published 2023 by John Wiley & Sons Ltd.

Rheumatoid arthritis (RA) is an autoimmune inflammatory disease that primarily affects synovial joints, such as hands, feet, and wrists. It is classically a symmetrical, peripheral inflammatory arthritis of an unknown origin. Although hands, feet, and wrists are the common sites, it can affect other parts of the body for example the lungs, heart, nervous system, kidneys, skin, and eyes. Extra articular features like anaemia, pericarditis, and hepatomegaly are also present. The immune system serves a vital protective role in the body and is triggered when something "foreign" enters the body, and complicated processes are initiated to eliminate it. However, in an autoimmune disorder, the immune system reacts against the body's own tissues. The body recognises its own tissues as " "foreign" and fights against itself. The risk of developing RA increases with age, commonly presenting between the ages of 30 to 50 years. Pre-menopausal women are more susceptible than men, in a 3:1 ratio. In some individuals, genetic factors are a crucial determinant of RA susceptibility. Tissue inflammation may occur due to persistent or exaggerated immune responses as a reaction to an infection or another challenge. Genetic factors are estimated to account for approximately 60% of susceptibility to the disease. There is an increased incidence of the disease among first-degree relatives. Environmental factors or triggers, such as obesity, smoking, and drinking, can increase the risk of developing RA in some individuals. Severe infections and traumatic events are also deemed significant to the development of RA.

Pathophysiology

RA is characterised by inflammation of the synovial lining of the joint capsule and increased synovial exudate, leading to thickening of the synovium and joint swelling. It is further characterised by exacerbation and remission of disease activity. Congestion occurs within the affected joints, accompanied by the presence of T lymphocytes, B cells, macrophages, and plasma cells. As the disease progresses, there is a gradual thickening of the lining forming a pannus, which then invades the articular cartilage and causes erosion of the cartilage and bone (Figure 46.1).

Presentation and clinical features

Classically, individuals present with symmetrical pain and swelling in the affected joints. Anaemia is a frequent extra-articular feature of RA, which can take several forms, but usually, it is normocytic and normochromic. This can be due to the excessive uptake of iron by the reticuloendothelial system. Early morning stiffness is a troublesome feature and is used as part of the assessment of disease activity. Inactivity stiffness occurs due to resting or sitting for extended periods. Pain and stiffness experienced can result in a loss of mobility and difficulty with rising and sitting or using aids due to for example, affected wrists. People also report feelings of general malaise, flu-like symptoms, tiredness, and fatigue. Fatigue is a predominant feature, and rest does not alleviate it. This can lead to irritability, anxiety, and depression. Some patients may experience weight loss, as acute and chronic inflammatory disease can increase the rate of metabolism, leading to energy expenditure exceeding dietary intake. Reduced mobility due to RA can also lead to weight gain, putting additional stress on affected joints. The pain, fatigue, and stiffness caused by RA can have social and psychological impacts on a person's daily activities at home, work, and socially. Family relationships may become stronger or weaker under the strain of coping with this long-term condition.

Common Co-Morbidities

People with RA are at a higher risk of several conditions, including cardiovascular disease. Around 6% of individuals with RA have cardiovascular disease, and they are twice as likely to have a heart attack and have a 30% higher risk of stroke compared to the general population. Lung disease is a significant contributor to morbidity and mortality in RA. The occurrence of osteoporosis can be up to twice as high in individuals with RA compared to the general population. People with RA are at a higher risk of falls, with a two-fold increased risk of hip fracture, and the risk of vertebral fractures is 2.4.

Diagnosis

Diagnosis of RA requires a comprehensive clinical examination, which includes blood tests and other investigations such as a full blood count (FBC), urea and electrolytes (U&Es), liver function tests (LFTs), erythrocyte sedimentation rate (ESR), C-reactive protein (CRP), anti-cyclic citrullinated peptide, plasma viscosity, rheumatoid factor (RF), MRI scans, X-rays, and joint aspiration. The growing body of knowledge regarding environmental and genetic factors is also taken into consideration.

Management

Rheumatoid arthritis exhibits classic characteristics that can manifest differently in various individuals. Prior to discussing and determining a medication regime with the patient, factors such as duration of illness, clinical presentation, and results of different investigations are considered. Medication can be prescribed in isolation or combination depending on the severity of symptoms and investigation findings. Although there is a range of medication available that cannot cure RA, it can slow down disease progression and minimise joint damage. The objective is to suppress inflammation as soon as possible to impede joint erosion, reduce symptoms, and manage the disease. These medications necessitate close monitoring due to the possibility of side effects (Table 46.1). Many individuals with RA can pinpoint dietary triggers that exacerbate their condition. Despite weak evidence concerning diet, adhering to healthy eating and Mediterranean diet principles is promoted. Encouraging and empowering individuals to manage their condition themselves is crucial and backed by solid evidence. The multidisciplinary team plays a vital role in providing care. NICE has issued a guideline on "depression in adults with chronic physical health problems." Voluntary organisations such as the National Rheumatoid Arthritis Society (NRAS) also offer support such as helpline assistance, education, and local group services. Communicating with other individuals with RA and sharing experiences helps individuals to realise that they are not alone.

Sickle cell

Barry Hill

Figure 47.1 Sickle cell. Source: Figure 10.8 from Peate (2022) Fundamentals of Applied Pathophysiology, Wiley, 4e, p. 275.

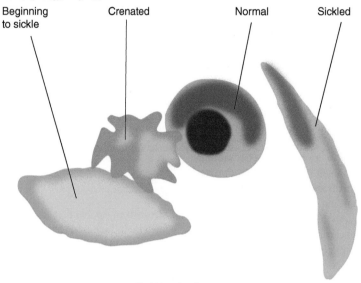

Beginning to sickle   Crenated   Normal   Sickled

Red blood cells

Table 47.1 Treatment of sickling episodes.

Most people who have a sickle cell crisis do not need to be admitted to hospital for treatment. If the pain is mild and there is no fever, then it can be possible to be treated at home. Treatment usually involves:
- Analgesia to prevent pain.
- Hydration to maintain adequate perfusion.
- Oxygen maybe required for hypoxia as this may cause red cells to become more sickle-shaped.
- Antibiotics to treat infection.
- Blood transfusion to correct anaemia and reduce the effects of sickling. There are potential side-effects from blood transfusions. Therefore, transfusions are given for a specific need, rather than routinely.
- Treatment of acute chest syndrome includes painkillers, hydration, and antibiotics, and potential blood transfusion and oxygen administration.
- Hydroxycarbamide (also called hydroxyurea) will reduce pain episodes and acute chest syndrome. Hydroxycarbamide can have serious side-effects and needs monitoring with blood tests.

Sickle cell disease (SCD) is a group of inherited red blood cell (RBC) disorders that affects haemoglobin, the protein that carries oxygen through the body. Most people affected are of African or African-Caribbean origin, although the sickle gene is found in all ethnic groups. SCD has a significant impact on morbidity and mortality. The recent advent of the COVID-19 pandemic has presented further concerns for this patient group and therefore it is imperative that health-care professionals have some knowledge and understanding about this important disease. SCD is the name for a group of inherited health conditions that affect the RBCs. The most serious type is called sickle cell anaemia.

Sickle cell anaemia is a genetic disorder, where abnormal haemoglobin in RBCs occurs due oxygen content of blood being lower than normal and results in the haemoglobin becoming sharp and sickle-shaped, instead of the doughnut shape. The deformed, crescent shape and stiff erythrocytes collapse easily and would dam up in small blood vessels, causing an interference with oxygen delivery. In the event of a crisis, people with sickle cell anaemia would experience extreme respiratory distress and excruciating pain, requiring pharmacological interventions including primary analgesic treatments such as non-steroidal anti-inflammatory drugs (NSAIDs), strong opioids, corticosteroids and low molecular heparin dose.

During an acute painful sickle cell episode, evidence from studies indicate that patients perceived a lack of monitoring of their pain and their vital signs. Inherited blood disorders such as thalassaemia can also cause decreased haemoglobin production. There are two main types of thalassaemia, alpha thalassaemia and beta thalassaemia.

Epidemiology

SCD is an autosomal, recessively inherited condition affecting the structure of haemoglobin. The UK National Screening Committee (UK NSC) recommends that all eligible pregnant women are offered screening for sickle cell and thalassaemia. Screening recommendations also extend to include blood spot screening of newborn babies. Approximately 15 000 people in the UK have SCD, and approximately one in 79 babies born in the UK carry sickle cell trait.

SCD, which is present in affected individuals at birth, causes the production of abnormal Hb. SDS is one of the most common inherited conditions worldwide, with over 300 000 children born with the condition each year globally, three-quarters of whom are born in Africa. The prevalence of SCD varies considerably across different ethnic communities, predominantly affecting people of African or African–Caribbean origin. Owing to population migration, SCD is now of increasing importance worldwide and there are increasing numbers of affected individuals in Europe and the United States. Within Europe, the UK has the largest population with the condition. In the UK it is estimated that there are 15 000 affected individuals, and approximately 300 infants born with the condition each year.

Pathogenesis

Haemoglobin (Hb) is a chromoprotein, found in RBCs and is composed of haem, which holds iron within its centre and globin, (a type of protein), composed of two different pairs of globin chains. Figure 47.1 illustrates the structure of the haemoglobin. There are over 600 million haemoglobin molecules in each RBC and the function of haemoglobin is to transport oxygen from the lungs to tissues and carbon dioxide from the tissues to the lungs for gaseous exchange.

Pathophysiology

Normally, the haemoglobin protein, which resides inside RBCs, attaches to oxygen in the lungs and carries it to all parts of the body. Healthy RBCs are flexible so that they can move through the smallest blood vessels. In SCD, the Hb is abnormal, causing the RBCs to be rigid and shaped like a 'C' or sickle, the shape from which the disease takes its name. Sickle cells can get stuck and block blood flow, causing pain and infections. Complications of SCD occur because the sickled cells block blood flow to specific organs. The worst complications include stroke, acute chest syndrome (a condition that lowers the level of oxygen in the blood), end organ damage, and in some cases premature death. For a child to inherit SCD, both parents must have either SCD (two sickle cell genes) or sickle cell trait (one sickle cell gene). There are variations of SCD called sickle C or sickle thalassaemia, which are serious conditions but are sometimes less severe.

Signs and symptoms

Symptoms of SCD come in episodes. The reason that symptoms come and go is that the RBCs can behave normally for much of the time – but if something makes too many of them sickle, the sickle cells cause symptoms. If there are severe and sudden symptoms due to sickling, this is called a sickle cell crisis.

Episodes of pain

These are also called a pain crisis or a vaso-occlusive crisis. They occur when sickle cells block small blood vessels in bones, which causes pain. Pain usually occurs in bones and joints. The pain can vary from mild to severe and may come on suddenly. A common symptom in babies and young children is when small bones in the fingers and toes become swollen and painful – this is known as dactylitis. Episodes of abdominal pain can occur if sickle cells block blood vessels in the abdomen.

Acute chest syndrome

This occurs when there are blocked blood vessels in the lungs and can sometimes occur with a lung infection. The symptoms can include chest pain, fever and shortness of breath. Babies and young children may have more vague symptoms and look generally unwell, be lethargic, be restless or have increased respiratory rate. Acute chest syndrome is very serious and, if it is suspected, people should be treated urgently in hospital. Acute chest syndrome can start a few days after a painful sickle crisis. It is most common in women who are pregnant or who have recently had a baby.

Infections

People with SCD are more prone to severe infections, particularly from certain types of bacteria, which can cause pneumonia, meningitis, septicaemia or bone infections. These include the pneumococcal, *Haemophilus influenzae* type b and meningococcal bacteria, and salmonella bacteria which can infect bones. Symptoms of infection include fever, feeling generally ill, and pain in the affected part of the body.

Treatment of sickling episodes can be seen in Table 47.1.

48 Schizophrenia

Reuben Pearce and Helen Robson

Table 48.1 Essential diagnostic requirements for schizophrenia (WHO 2019).

Persistent delusions	Grandiose delusions, delusions of reference, persecutory delusions.
Persistent hallucinations	Most commonly auditory, although they may be in any sensory modality.
Disorganised thinking (Formal thought disorder)	Tangentiality and loose associations, irrelevant speech, neologisms. When severe, the person's speech may be so incoherent as to be incomprehensible.
Experiences of influence, passivity of control	The experience that one's feelings, impulses, actions, or thoughts are not generated by oneself, are being placed in one's mind or withdrawn from one's mind by others, or that one's thoughts are being broadcast to others.
Negative symptoms	Affective flattening, alogia or paucity of speech, avolition, asociality and anhedonia.
Grossly disorganised behaviour that impedes goal-directed activity	Behaviour that appears bizarre or purposeless, unpredictable, or inappropriate emotional responses that interfere with the ability to organise behaviour.
Psycho-motor disturbances	Catatonic restlessness or agitation, posturing, waxy flexibility, negativism, mutism, or stupor.

Schizophrenia is a psychotic disorder that includes a collection of psychotic symptoms, and can be described as the most severe form of the psychotic disorders. In addition, it is highly changeable in how symptoms present. Schizophrenia is characterised by changes in a person's perception, disordered thoughts, and social withdrawal.

Schizophrenia usually develops during the late teens or early twenties and males will often develop symptoms earlier than females. It is not uncommon for males to go on to develop a more serious illness. Schizophrenia in children under 18 is very rare. Earlier onset of schizophrenia is likely to lead to a more severe, harder-to-treat condition, however, early intervention can make a huge difference to prognosis. Delusional symptoms tend to be more evident than perceptual disturbances and social withdrawal.

There is often a prodromal phase ahead of someone developing schizophrenia. In the prodromal phase a person may present with non-specific, non-diagnosable thoughts, feelings, and behaviours. People close to them such as family members may report a change such as social withdrawal, lack of interest in usual activities, mood changes, and periods of unexplained confusion or distraction. These symptoms will usually be described as a change to the healthy state of that person.

There can be many reasons beyond the prodromal period of schizophrenia for the changes in a person just described, however, it is important to be aware and to work with a person and their family to monitor and over time formulate what is happening to inform the required medical treatment and psycho-social interventions.

Symptoms

The symptoms of schizophrenia are split between positive symptoms which can be described as something added to the usual functioning of a person and negative symptoms which can be described as something taken away from the usual functioning of a person.

Positive symptoms

Positive symptoms in schizophrenia are delusions and hallucinations. A delusion can be described as an unshakable false belief. The belief would unlikely be a usual part of a person's spiritual, cultural, subculture or social norms and would be deemed extremely unlikely to be true by others. If challenged on a delusional belief a person may be very defensive. Delusions are often persecutory which means a person may feel people are trying to cause them harm, blame, control or take things away from them. This can be very distressing for the individual and those around them.

Hallucinations are a disturbance of perception that can be described as experiences and sensations that are not apparent to others. The hallucination will seem real to the person experiencing them. Hallucinations can affect any of the five senses, sight (visual), hearing (auditory), touch (tactile), smell (olfactory), and taste (gustatory). People with schizophrenia are most likely to experience auditory hallucinations of one or more voices talking in the third person commenting on them. However, people may also experience hallucinations in any one or more of the other senses.

Negative symptoms

Negative symptoms are functions that become deficit in an individual with schizophrenia and can include impairment or loss of volition, motivation, and spontaneous behaviour. It is also common to see a loss of awareness of socially appropriate behaviour and social withdrawal. Those around that person may see a flattening of mood, blunting of affect (diminished expression of emotions) and anhedonia which is the inability to feel pleasure. People with schizophrenia may present through poverty of thought and speech due to a loss to their normal flow of thinking. Other symptoms may include features of depressive or manic mood, or psycho-motor features such as catatonia and cognitive impairment.

Diagnosis

To be diagnosed with schizophrenia, the ICD-11 (World Health Organization 2019) suggests at least two essential symptoms must be present (Table 48.1), including positive, negative, depressive, manic, psycho-motor, and cognitive symptoms. Of the two symptoms, one is be persistent delusions, hallucinations, disorganised thinking, or experience of passivity of control (Table 48.1). Symptoms should have been present for most of the time during a period of at least one month. The symptoms must not be a manifestation of another health condition such as brain tumour and not because of a substance or medication effect on the central nervous system.

Prevalence

Prevalence of schizophrenia is consistent worldwide with approximately a 1% lifetime risk of developing the condition across the population. There is no research that has been able to provide an exact cause of schizophrenia, however, evidence suggests that a mixture of physical, genetic, psychological, and environmental factors may contribute to an individual being more susceptible to developing the condition. There is evidence to suggest stressful life events may trigger someone who is susceptible to developing schizophrenia.

Genetics

There does appear to be some evidence of genetic factors with risk percentages of 46% in identical twins, 40% when both parents had the condition, up to 25% when one parent had the condition, 12–15% sibling and 6% grandparent. When no relative has been affected the risk is reduced to 0.5–1%, so there is a significant difference (Coelewij and Curtis 2018).

Brain and chemical differences

There are also studies of people with schizophrenia which have shown that there are subtle differences in the structure of their brains. These changes are not seen in everyone with schizophrenia and can occur in people who do not have a mental illness. There is some evidence suggesting childbirth complications may contribute to people developing schizophrenia such as a low birthweight, premature labour, and starvation of oxygen during birth which could influence brain development.

It has also been identified that there may be differing levels of the serotonin and dopamine neurotransmitters which carry messages between brain cells which may contribute to negative and positive symptoms of schizophrenia.

Mortality

Premature mortality is very high for people with schizophrenia and tragically they will on average die 20–25 years earlier than the wider population. There are several factors that are believed to contribute relating to lifestyle, physical health factors, access to health care and socioeconomic issues. However, suicide is the most common cause of early death (38%) of people with schizophrenia.

Support, treatment and relapse prevention

The National Institute for Health and Care Excellence (2014) guidance on psychosis and schizophrenia suggest that support and treatment of someone with schizophrenia needs to be person-centred and tailored to meet the individual needs of the person and their family/carers. Care needs to be holistic, addressing the biological, psychological, social and spiritual factors that impact on a person's chances of recovery.

Anti-psychotic medication can be used to reduce symptoms, however, needs careful monitoring due to unpleasant side-effects which impact on physical health such as weight gain and movement disorders. Counter measures may need to be agreed with the patient to mitigate some of the side-effects of anti-psychotics such as nutrition planning, exercise, and other lifestyle changes.

Psycho-education is important to aid a person and their family in understanding the illness and the steps to take to maintain good health with agreed warning signs. Steps to take should there be signs of deterioration are important for relapse prevention.

Psycho-social interventions such as cognitive behavioural therapy and art therapy can be useful in helping somebody to understand better and cope with their symptoms. Family interventions can be useful for shared understanding within the family and help to manage relationships.

49 Vascular dementia

Ian Peate

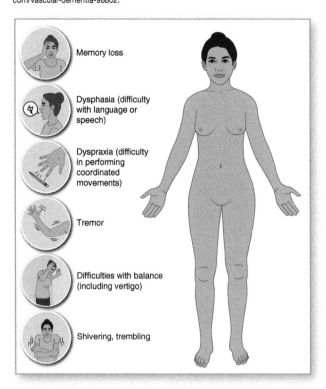

Figure 49.1 Vascular dementia symptoms. From: www.verywellhealth. com/vascular-dementia-98802.

Memory loss

Dysphasia (difficulty with language or speech)

Dyspraxia (difficulty in performing coordinated movements)

Tremor

Difficulties with balance (including vertigo)

Shivering, trembling

Table 49.1 Symptoms related to specific subtypes of dementia.

Subtype	Symptoms
Alzheimer's disease	Presenting symptom is usually loss of recent memory first and often difficulty with executive function and/or nominal dysphasia. Loss of episodic memory. This may include memory loss for recent events, repeated questioning and difficulty learning new information. Cognitive deficits can include aphasia, apraxia and agnosia.
Vascular dementia	Step by step increases in the severity of symptoms, may present insidiously with gait and attention problems and changes in personality. Focal neurological signs (hemiparesis or visual field defects) may be present.
Dementia with Lewy bodies	Core clinical features are fluctuating cognition; recurrent visual hallucinations, sleep behaviour disorder and one or more symptoms of parkinsonism, bradykinesia, rest tremor or rigidity. Memory impairment in early stages may not be apparent.
Frontotemporal dementia	Personality change and behavioural disturbance (apathy or social/sexual disinhibition) may develop insidiously. Other cognitive functions (memory and perception) may be relatively preserved.

Dementia

This condition is a progressive, irreversible clinical syndrome that is accompanied by a variety of cognitive and behavioural symptoms. The symptoms include memory loss, problems with reasoning and communication, change in personality and a reduction in the individual's capacity to perform daily activities.

The decline in cognition is extensive, often affecting multiple domains of intellectual functioning; this impairment is not entirely attributable to normal ageing.

For a diagnosis of dementia to be made, the person must have impairment in at least two of the following cognitive domains: memory, language, behaviour, visuospatial or executive function. These impairments have to cause a substantial functional decline

Long-term Conditions in Adults at a Glance, First Edition. Edited by Aby Mitchell, Barry Hill, and Ian Peate.
© 2023 John Wiley & Sons Ltd. Published 2023 by John Wiley & Sons Ltd.

in their usual activities or work. The impairments cannot be explained by delirium or other major psychiatric disorder.

Causes of dementia

The majority of causes of dementia are a result of neurodegenerative diseases.

- Alzheimer's disease is responsible for most cases of dementia; it often co-exists with other forms of dementia, for example, vascular dementia. Young-onset Alzheimer's disease, in some people, has a genetic cause.
- Vascular dementia is the second most common type of dementia, occurring as a result of reduced blood supply to the brain. Young-onset vascular dementia has a genetic cause in some people.
- Dementia with Lewy bodies is a common cause of dementia in the older person.
- Frontotemporal dementia is being increasingly recognised as a common cause of dementia, particularly in younger people. A significant proportion of people, particularly those with behavioural presentations, have a family history. Onset of frontotemporal dementia is typically in the sixth decade of life, but it can be as early as the third or as late as the ninth decade.

Dementia: clinical features

It can be difficult to identify dementia as it often has an insidious onset with non-specific signs and symptoms; these vary from person to person. Those with early dementia may refute any symptoms or they will accommodate to cognitive change and functional ability. If any of the following are reported by the person and/or their family/carer then dementia should be suspected:

- There may be cognitive impairment, including memory loss.
- The person may defer to family when they are answering questions.
- They may have difficulty learning new information or remembering recent events or people's names.
- They can be vague with dates, and/or miss appointments.
- There may be problems with reasoning and communication, difficulty in making decisions, dysphasia, and challenges when undertaking coordinated movements, for example, dressing.
- There may be disorientation and unawareness of time and place.
- There may be impairment of executive function, such as difficulties with planning, judgement, loss of initiative and problem-solving.

Behavioural and psychological symptoms of dementia tend to fluctuate; they may last for six months or more and include psychosis, or the person may have delusions (persecutory) and/or hallucinations (visual and auditory). The person may be easily upset, argumentative, shout, have mood swings and/or exhibit physically and verbally challenging behaviour (agitation and emotional lability). The onset of depression in later life is a warning sign of dementia. They may be withdrawn or apathetic. The person may display socially or sexually inappropriate behaviour, they may wander, become restless, pace and perform repetitive activity. Sleep cycle disturbance or insomnia can occur. There is a tendency to repeat phrases or questions. In the early stages of dementia this may lead to difficulty carrying out complex household tasks. In the later stages, undertaking basic activities of living, including bathing, toileting, eating and walking can become affected.

See Figure 49.1, neurological and cognitive symptoms and also Table 49.1 for symptoms related to specific subtypes of dementia.

Diagnosis

An initial assessment and a history is undertaken from the person and, if possible, from someone who knows the person well, for example, a family member. When taking a history from someone who knows the person with suspected dementia, if possible supplement this with a structured questionnaire. The person's current level of cognition and functional capabilities should be compared to their baseline level helping to detect whether there has been a significant decline. Appropriate blood tests are taken to exclude reversible causes of cognitive decline.

Vascular dementia

Dementia describes a set of symptoms including memory loss and difficulties with thinking, problem-solving or language. In vascular dementia, these symptoms arise when the supply of blood to the brain is impeded. The death of brain cells as a result of hindered blood supply can cause problems with cognition. When these cognitive problems occur they can have a substantial impact on daily life. There are different types of vascular dementia, they have some symptoms in common and symptoms that differ.

Stroke-related dementia

Strokes vary in how severe they are, depending on where the blocked vessel is and whether the interruption to the blood supply is permanent or temporary. Not everyone who has a stroke will develop vascular dementia, but about 20% of people who have a stroke do develop this post-stroke dementia within the following six months. A person who has a stroke is then at increased risk of having further strokes. If this happens, the risk of developing dementia is higher.

Single-infarct and multi-infarct dementia

These types of vascular dementia are caused by one or more smaller strokes occurring when a large or medium-sized blood vessel is blocked by a clot. The stroke may be so small that the person does not notice any symptoms (transient ischaemic attack). If the blood supply is interrupted for more than a few minutes, the stroke will lead to brain cell death (cerebral infarct). There can be many cerebral infarcts; dementia in this case is caused by the total damage from all the infarcts together.

Subcortical dementia

Subcortical vascular dementia is caused by diseases of the very small blood vessels deep in the brain. These small vessels develop thick walls, becoming stiff and tortuous; blood flow through them is reduced. Small vessel disease often damages the bundles of nerve fibres that transmit signals throughout the brain, known as white matter. It can also result in small infarcts near the base of the brain. Small vessel disease develops much deeper in the brain than the damage caused by many strokes. The symptoms of subcortical vascular dementia are therefore different from those of stroke-related dementia. Subcortical dementia is thought to be the most common type of vascular dementia.

Mixed dementia (vascular dementia and Alzheimer's disease)

Generally, this means that both Alzheimer's disease and vascular disease are thought to have caused the dementia. The symptoms of mixed dementia may be similar to those of either Alzheimer's disease or vascular dementia or they could be a combination of the two.

Viral hepatitis

50

Ian Peate

Table 50.1   A summary of the hepatitides.

Hepatitide	Discussion
A (HAV)	Acquired by ingesting contaminated water or food or having close contact with an infected person or their waste (faecal–oral route). No specific treatment, majority of patients recover fully and have life-long immunity afterward. A minority can develop life-threatening acute liver failure. Safe and effective vaccine available to prevent HAV. Symptoms include fatigue, nausea, diarrhoea, abdominal pain, loss of appetite fever or jaundice.
B (HBV)	Transmitted through direct exposure to infected bodily fluids through contaminated needles, sexual partners or between family members. Pregnant mothers can transmit HBV to newborns during birth. HBV can directly cause liver cancer in the absence of cirrhosis. Currently, antiviral therapies control chronic HBV infections by stopping viral production. Safe and effective HBV vaccines are available. Symptoms include fatigue, abdominal pain, jaundice, or dark-coloured urine.
C (HCV)	Spread through direct exposure to blood or bodily fluids. Can be transmitted from a mother to newborn. Acute infection resolves spontaneously in a minority of people; however the majority develop chronic HCV that normally progresses over many years. Once chronic HCV progresses to cirrhosis, liver cancer risk increases. Absence of symptoms leads to progressive liver damage before the person becomes aware of their infection. Symptoms at that time may include, fatigue, poor appetite, jaundice or dark-coloured urine, easy bruising, oedema, ascites or gastrointestinal bleeding. Currently, no vaccine available; however there are very effective treatments available for HCV with direct acting antiviral medications.
D (HDV)	HDV only infects people with HBV infection, as the HDV life cycle depends on HBV proteins. A dual HDV and HBV infection increases severity of liver injury and the pace of progression to cirrhosis. Symptoms are similar to those in patients with HBV infection. All patients with HBV infection should be tested for HDV infection. Vaccine prevention of HBV infection eliminates the risk of HDV infection.
E (HEV)	HEV infection, like HAV results from ingestion of contaminated food and water. HEV infection generally resolves spontaneously, however, in pregnant women it may result in acute liver failure and death. HEV infection may not resolve spontaneously in those with compromised immune systems. Symptoms are similar to those in HAV infection. Antiviral medications can cure chronic HEV infection.

Table 50.2   Hepatitis at a glance.

Name of virus	Hepatitis A virus (HAV)	Hepatitis B virus (HBV)	Hepatitis C virus (HCV)	Hepatitis D virus (HDV)	Hepatitis E virus (HEV)
Transmission	Enteric	Parental	Parental	Parental	Enteric
Incubation period	15–45 d	45–160 d	15–150 d	30–60 d	15–60 d
Chronic hepatitis	No.	Yes. 10% chance	Yes. >50% chance	Yes. <5% of coinfectious >80% of superinfectious	No
Cure?	No cure. Treatments usually tackle the symptoms.	No cure. Treatments usually tackle the symptoms.	No cure. Treatments usually tackle the symptoms.	No cure. Treatment: Alpha interferon for 12 months.	No cure. Treatments usually tackle the symptoms.

Long-term Conditions in Adults at a Glance, First Edition. Edited by Aby Mitchell, Barry Hill, and Ian Peate.
© 2023 John Wiley & Sons Ltd. Published 2023 by John Wiley & Sons Ltd.

Hepatitis

Inflammation of the liver is called hepatitis. When sudden inflammation of the liver occurs (acute hepatitis) and if the liver remains inflamed for months or years, this is a chronic long-term condition called hepatitis. Viral hepatitis is inflammation of the liver as a result of a viral infection. It is most commonly caused by hepatitis A, B, C, and E.

If left untreated, there are some types of viral hepatitis that can cause liver damage, resulting in scarring and necrosis. Scar tissue (cirrhosis) can, over time prevent the liver from performing effectively. In severe cases, liver failure or liver cancer can occur.

Hepatitis A

Globally, Hepatitis A is the most common viral hepatitis. It can be acquired in various ways. Transmission for most people is through eating food or drinking water which has been contaminated with infected faeces as a result of poor hygiene or inadequate cooking (the faecal–oral route). These infections can, less commonly, be transmitted through cuts in the skin or mucous membranes. Common risk factors are through sharing razor blades, toothbrushes or needles if injecting drugs. Hepatitis A can be also passed on by having unprotected sex with a person who already has the virus. It presents with nausea, vomiting, anorexia and jaundice. It can cause cholestasis with dark urine and pale stools and moderate hepatomegaly. It resolves without treatment in around one to three months. Vaccination is available to reduce the chance of developing the infection. It is a notifiable disease and Public Health need to be notified of all cases.

Hepatitis B

Hepatitis B is transmitted by direct contact with blood or bodily fluids, such as during sexual intercourse or sharing needles (intravenous drug users or tattoos). It can also be transmitted through sharing contaminated household products, for example, toothbrushes or contact between minor cuts or abrasions. It can also be passed from mother to child during pregnancy and delivery (vertical transmission). This virus cannot be transmitted through food or water or 'casual' contact, such as holding hands, coughing or sneezing.

Most people fully recover from the infection within two months, however around 10% will go on to become chronic hepatitis B carriers. In these patients the virus DNA has integrated into their own DNA and as such they will continue to produce the viral proteins.

Vaccination is available and this involves injecting the hepatitis B surface antigen. Vaccinated patients are tested for hepatitis B surface antibody (HBsAb) to confirm their response to the vaccine. The vaccine requires three doses at different intervals. Vaccination to hepatitis B is now included as part of the UK routine vaccination schedule (as part of the six in one vaccine).

Hepatitis C

Transmission occurs via contaminated blood. Common risk factors include sharing contaminated needles during intravenous drug use, sharing personal items that are contaminated with blood, for example, razors or having unprotected sex with someone who already has the virus. It can be transmitted from mother to baby during birth. Previously people have been infected with hepatitis C via blood products although these are now thoroughly tested in the UK and are safe. Currently, there is no vaccine available; however there are very effective treatments available for hepatitis C with direct acting antiviral medications. One in four people fight off the virus and make a full recovery, for three in four it becomes a long-term condition. Complications include cirrhosis and associated complications and hepatocellular carcinoma.

Hepatitis D

This virus can only survive in patients who also have a hepatitis B infection. The virus attaches itself to the HBsAg to survive and is unable to survive without this protein. There are very low rates in the UK. Hepatitis D increases the complications and disease severity of hepatitis B. There is no specific treatment for hepatitis D and there is no vaccine, but if a person been vaccinated against hepatitis B this also protects them from hepatitis D. It is a notifiable disease and Public Health need to be notified of all cases.

Hepatitis E

Like hepatitis A, hepatitis E is transmitted by the faecal–oral route. It is very rare in the UK. Normally it produces only a mild illness and the virus is cleared within a month and no treatment is needed. Rarely it can progress to chronic hepatitis and liver failure, this occurs more in those patients who are immunocompromised. There is no vaccination for hepatitis E. It is a notifiable disease and Public Health need to be notified of all cases.

See Table 50.1 for a summary of the hepatitides. Table 50.2 provides an overview of hepatitis at a glance.

Supporting people with viral hepatitis

People with hepatitis should be diagnosed as early as possible and if they are at risk of preventable liver disease they should be offered preventative advice. A detailed assessment is undertaken and the relevant care pathway followed. Appropriate referral to other health and care professionals may be required (hepatologist, gastroenterologist). Advice should be offered about how to reduce the risk of developing liver disease, such as eating a healthy diet, losing weight, increasing exercise and reducing alcohol intake to no more than the Government's recommended amount.

A number of visits to specialist clinicians may be needed as well as a number of tests so as to make a specific diagnosis. An opportunity must be provided for the patient (and if appropriate family) to discuss any concerns. If a diagnosis of hepatitis is made the patient must be provided with information and advice.

The person should be able to discuss the cause of illness in a way that is free from stigma and prejudice, be provided with plenty of time to ask questions, have their concerns listened to and their wishes respected. Support should be offered so that the person can manage their condition as far as possible, so that they and their family can continue to lead an independent life.

It should be determined whether additional support such as access to a social worker, counselling or information about benefits and financial support are needed. It should be ensured that care is properly coordinated by a multi-disciplinary team.

Being diagnosed with a long-term condition requires that the person's treatment should be tailored to their condition and their situation, including emotional, physical, practical and spiritual care. Well-coordinated supportive care comes about when the patient is at the centre of all that is done and the health and care provider are knowledgeable and aware of the needs of those with viral hepatitis.

51 Visual impairment

Caitlin Gallon and Claire Ford

Table 51.1 Common eye conditions that can cause visual impairment (NICE 2022, RNIB 2014a,b, and Bainter 2019).

Condition	Description	Symptoms	Diagnostics	Treatment
Age-related macular degeneration (AMD)	• AMD causes changes to the macula, a part of the retina at the back of the eye. • There are two types of AMD, wet AMD, and dry AMD, both cause problems with central vision. • AMD does not affect peripheral vision; therefore, the condition does not result in complete blindness.	• Reduced vision. • Detail and small print are often harder to see. • Distorted and blurry central vision. • Straight lines appear wavy. • Blank patches may appear in the central vision. • Increased sensitivity to light.	• Visual acuity test • Dilated fundus exam • Optical coherence tomography (OCT)	• Anti-VEGF injections for Wet AMD. These medications reduce new blood vessel growth. • There is currently no treatment for dry AMD. However, there is some evidence that high doses of certain antioxidant, vitamins, such as C and E, can slow down the progression of dry AMD.
Cataract	• A cataract is a term associated with the lens of the eye becoming cloudy. • They normally appear in both eyes, but often at different times. • They are usually age-related and most common in individuals over 65 years of age. • Cataracts can also be congenital and affect babies and young children.	• Eyesight is misty and cloudy. • Increased sensitivity to light and bright sunlight. • Car headlamps may glare more than usual. • Vision appears more washed-out.	• Visual acuity test • Dilated fundus exam	• Cataracts can only be removed by surgery, which involves the removal of the cloudy lens that is replaced with a permanent artificial lens. • The artificial lens is made of plastic or silicone and usually lasts for the lifetime of the individual.

Glaucoma	• Glaucoma is caused when the optic nerve, which connects the eye to the brain, becomes damaged. As a result, fluid increases at the front part of the eye and intraocular pressure rises because the fluid can't drain through the trabecular meshwork.
	• Glaucoma affects peripheral vision over time, and without treatment, can lead to blindness.
	• There are several types of glaucoma:
	  ○ Primary open-angle glaucoma
	  ○ Acute closed-angle glaucoma
	  ○ Secondary glaucoma
	  ○ Congenital glaucoma (children).
		• Early glaucoma is often asymptotic.
		• Late symptoms often include:
		  ○ Blurred vision
		  ○ Seeing rainbow-coloured circles around bright lights
		• If glaucoma occurs suddenly (i.e. due to medication or trauma) it is usually associated with:
		  ○ Intense pain
		  ○ Nausea and vomiting
		  ○ Headache
		  ○ Blurred vision
		  ○ Tenderness around the eyes.
			• Visual acuity test
			• Visual fields test
			• OCT of the optic nerve
			• Dilated fundus exam
			• Intraocular pressure examination
				• Eye drops containing a generic prostaglandin analogue (PGA) can be used to reduce intraocular pressure.
				• 360° selective laser trabeculoplasty (SLT) can be used to clear debris from the trabecular meshwork, increasing the draining of fluid and reducing intraocular pressure.
				• Surgery involving electrocautery, or a trabeculectomy can also be used to drain fluid but are more invasive.

Diabetic retinopathy	• Diabetic retinopathy is a complication of diabetes (type 1 and 2). • The retina needs a constant supply of blood, but these blood vessels can become damaged, due to high blood sugar levels. • If left undiagnosed and untreated it can cause blindness.	• Reduced vision. • Sudden loss of vision. • Floating shapes in peripheral vision. • Patchy or blurred vision. • Red eyes and eye pain. • Reduced night vision.	• Visual acuity test • Dilated fundus exam • OCT	• Laser treatment • Anti-VEGF injections • Surgery: Vitrectomy surgery removes blood or scar tissue from the eye.

Long-term Conditions in Adults at a Glance, First Edition. Edited by Aby Mitchell, Barry Hill, and Ian Peate.
© 2023 John Wiley & Sons Ltd. Published 2023 by John Wiley & Sons Ltd.

Within the UK, is it estimated that over 2 million people live with sight loss severe enough to have a significant impact on their lives and every day 250 new people begin to lose their sight; that's one person every six minutes. Sight loss can affect individuals of all ages; however, it is more prevalent amongst the older generation and with the growing ageing population, it is predicted one in five individuals will experience sight loss in their lifetime.

The main causes of sight loss in the UK are diabetic retinopathy, glaucoma, age-related macular degeneration (AMD) and cataracts (see Table 51.1) and the general risk factors associated with sight loss include, obesity, hypertension, smoking, diabetes and a family history of eye disease. Consequently, it is paramount that health-care professionals make every contact count to promote eye health, by ensuring their patients attend regular optician appointments and maintain a healthy lifestyle. Current recommendations suggest that individuals should have their sight tested every two years; however, professionals may advise more regular testing for young children wearing glasses, individuals with diabetes, people aged over 40 with a family history of glaucoma and individuals over 70 years of age.

Eye function

The eye is a sense organ and part of the sensory nervous system. It sits within the orbit (is a pyramid-shaped cavity), is approximately 2.5 cm in diameter, spherical and supplied by the optic nerve (second cranial nerve). The eye wall consists of three layers, the inner layer is made up of the retina, the iris, ciliary body and choroid create the middle layer and the cornea and sclera form the outer layer.

Vision occurs when each part of the eye works together, culminating in the ability to create a perception of objects by the interpretation of electromagnetic. First, light enters the cornea, a transparent dome-like structure covering the front of the eye and responsible for refracting the light onto the lens as it enters the eye. Some of the light then enters the pupil which is the dark circular opening in the centre of the eye, controlled by the dilator and sphincter muscles of the iris. Depending on the intensity of light, the iris will either dilate or constrict the pupil to determine how much light enters through the pupil and is transmitted to the lens, a transparent circular structure enclosed within a thin capsule which sits directly behind the pupil. The remaining light then passes through the lens and vitreous until it reaches the retina at the back of the eye. The retina is the light-sensitive layer of the eye and contains photoreceptors constructed from cones and rods, which transform light into electrical impulses. These then travel along the optic nerve to the occipital lobe and the visual processing area of the brain.

Visual acuity

One of the most important parts of any ophthalmic assessment is an accurate assessment of visual acuity (VA). VA refers to an individual's ability to see small detail, but it is also used as it indicates the clarity and sharpness of vision. Other elements incorporated into the overall assessment of vision include colour vision, peripheral vision, near vision and depth perception and one of the most common tools used when testing distance VA is the Snellen chart. The chart displays letters or symbols in lines of diminishing size and each line is labelled with a number. VA is always tested monocularly whilst wearing glasses or contact lenses if a refractive error is present and the chart should be positioned approximately 6 m from the patient who read out the lowest line visible. The resulting VA scores obtained by the professional are usually written as a fraction; the numerator being the test distance in metres (usually 6) and the denominator the smallest line the patient was able to read, e.g. the third line from the top is recorded as 6/24 as their VA was tested at 6 m and they read to the line labelled 24. Any condition affecting the light pathway, such as a problem with the optic nerve, the lens, cornea, tear film, vitreous, retina, or the brain can lead to a reduced VA. Uncorrected refractive errors (myopia/hyperopia/astigmatism) are the most common cause of reduced visual acuity and are usually corrected with prescription glasses.

Pharmacology

The most common method of drug delivery to the eyes is topical eye drops or ointments, which are more effective than oral medications. They are usually prescribed to treat acute or long-term eye conditions such as infection, and inflammation and to relieve discomfort for patients with dry eye. For maximum therapeutic gain, it is vital that topical eye drops, and ointments are given the same priority as medications that are administered systemically. Compliance and poor administration technique are two of the main barriers associated with the administration of eye drops or ointments; however, physical barriers such as poor vision, arthritis and cognitive impairment can also hinder the effectiveness of drop administration. Therefore, it is essential that health-care professionals possess a comprehensive understanding of the therapeutic effects, drug interactions and side-effects of the prescribed treatment, and explain the rationale, administration technique and expected result to the patient or carer to reduce any potential barrier.

Management of long-term conditions

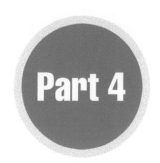

Part 4

Chapters

52 **Frameworks of care delivery – new ways of working** 120
53 **Evidence-based practice** 122
54 **Leadership and management** 124
55 **Chronic pain management** 126
56 **End of life care** 130
57 **Advanced care planning** 132

52 Frameworks of care delivery – new ways of working

Barry Hill

Table 52.1 Social care for older people with multiple long-term conditions.

Social care-related quality of life
Health-related quality of life
Involvement in decision-making
Safety of people using services
Hospital admissions
Residential care admissions
Older people being supported to live where they wish
Service user and carer satisfaction

Table 52.2 Three crucial gaps identified in the FYFV.

Health and well-being: Without a greater focus on prevention, health inequalities will widen and our capacity to pay for new treatments will be compromised by the need to spend billions of pounds on avoidable illness.

Care and quality: Health needs will go unmet unless we reshape care, harness technology and address variations in quality and safety.

Funding and efficiency: Without efficiencies, a shortage of resources will hinder care services and progress.

Figure 52.1 Leading change and adding value.

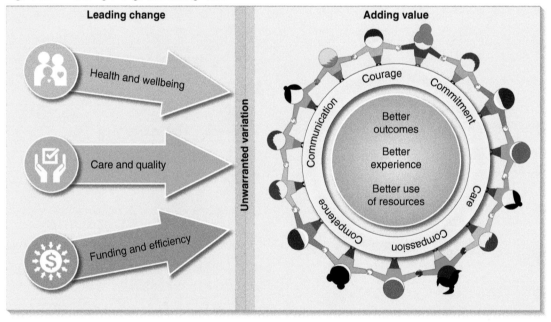

Long-term Conditions in Adults at a Glance, First Edition. Edited by Aby Mitchell, Barry Hill, and Ian Peate.
© 2023 John Wiley & Sons Ltd. Published 2023 by John Wiley & Sons Ltd.

Social care for older people with multiple long-term conditions

Older people with multiple long-term conditions are likely to have a wide range of care needs because of their conditions. Those with social care needs may need support with personal care and other practical assistance. Despite recent policy focusing on integrated health and social care services, some people are still treated as a collection of conditions or symptoms, rather than as a whole person, and there can be poor coordination of care. There is significant variability in the commissioning and provision of health and social care for people in England. Although good practice on integrating health and social care is beginning to emerge from local areas that have developed new approaches to transforming services, considerable variability remains. This quality standard has been developed in the context of important legal changes affecting people with social care needs. The Care Act 2014 establishes new provisions as well as updating existing ones, bringing together relevant policy and guidance that may have a significant impact on this group. The NICE quality standard for social care for older people with multiple long-term conditions is expected to contribute to improvements in several outcomes (Table 52.1).

Person-centred care framework

The person-centred care framework by Health Education England aids the development of workforce and community with behaviours, skills and competencies that support and drive person-centred approaches to well-being, prevention, care and support. Being person-centred is about focusing care on the needs of individuals. It is also noted that health professionals must ensure that people's preferences, needs, and values guide clinical decisions, and provide care that is respectful and responsive to their needs. Health and well-being outcomes need to be co-produced by individuals and members of the workforce working in partnership, with evidence suggesting that this provides better patient outcomes and costs less to health and care systems. The person-centred approach is a core skills education and training framework that articulates what it means to be person-centred and how to develop and support the workforce to work in this way. Developed in partnership with Skills for Health and Skills for Care, the Framework aims to distil best practice and to set out core, transferable behaviours, knowledge, and skills. It is applicable across services and sectors (e.g. health, social care, local authorities, and housing) and across different types of organisations (e.g. public, private and not for profit). Person-centred approaches underpin existing dementia, learning disabilities, mental health, and end-of-life care core skills frameworks. There are six principles that are aimed to support change of how behaviours and competencies can be developed to enable all people to sustain engagement, be healthy and in be in control of their own choices.

Leading change, adding value

Leading Change, Adding Value is a framework for all nursing, midwifery, and care staff, whatever their role or place of work (Figure 52.1). This framework builds upon Compassion in Practice and is directly aligned with the five-year forward view (FYFV) in seeking to develop new ways of working that are person-focused and provide seamless care across the boundary that has traditionally separated health and social care. It aims to target three crucial gaps identified in the FYFV. These are listed in Table 52.2.

Nursing, midwifery, and care staff have a crucial role to play in closing these gaps, by ensuring the activities we undertake are of high value. This framework aims to help achieve that by closing the health and well-being gap by practising in ways which prevent avoidable illness, protect health, and promote well-being and resilience. Closing the care and quality gap by practising in ways which provide safe evidence-based care maximises choice for patients. Closing the funding and efficiency gap by practising in ways which manage resources well including time, equipment, and referrals. The overall objective is to develop a high quality, financially sustainable service that delivers the objectives set out under using a triple aim in achieving: (i) better outcomes; (ii) better experiences; and (iii) better use of resources.

National framework for NHS continuing healthcare and NHS-funded nursing care

The revised 2022 National Framework for NHS Continuing Healthcare and NHS-funded Nursing Care sets out the principles and processes of NHS Continuing Healthcare and NHS-funded Nursing Care. This guidance replaces the previous version of the National Framework, published in March 2018, and was implemented in July 2022. It includes Practice Guidance to support staff delivering NHS Continuing Healthcare. This revised 2022 National Framework follows a period of engagement with stakeholders, across the NHS, Local Authorities, and patient representative groups. The 2022 National Framework has been collaboratively written by the Department of Health (DH), NHS England, and Local Authorities. The 2022 National Framework is intended to reflect legislative changes since the 2018 National Framework was published, primarily to incorporate the Health and Care Act 2022. This updated framework aimed to clarify several policy areas, including:

(i) Strengthening guidance which sets out that most NHS Continuing Healthcare assessments should take place outside of acute hospital settings. This will ensure alignment with current hospital discharge policy and reflects best practice around the 'Discharge to Assess' model.

(ii) Clarifying when consent and informed and active participation should be sought throughout the NHS Continuing Healthcare process.

(iii) Providing clearer guidance on 'best interests' decision-making in NHS Continuing Healthcare.

(iv) Providing additional advice on resolving interagency disputes, recognising the responsibilities and makeup of the new Integrated Care Boards.

53 Evidence-based practice

Claire Anderson

Figure 53.1   Hierarchy of evidence: a framework for evaluating health-care interventions. Source: https://onlinelibrary.wiley.com/doi/10.1046/j.1365-2702.2003.00662.x.

	Effectiveness	Appropriateness	Feasibility
Excellent	• Systematic review • Multi-centre studies	• Systematic review • Multi-centre studies	• Systematic review • Multi-centre studies
Good	• RCT • Observational studies	• RCT • Observational studies • Interpretive studies	• RCT • Observational studies • Interpretive studies
Fair	• Uncontrolled trials with dramatic results • Before and after studies • Non-randomized controlled trails	• Descriptive studies • Focus groups	• Descriptive studies • Action research • Before and after studies • Focus groups
Poor	• Descriptive studies • Case studies • Expert opinion • Studies of poor methodological quality	• Expert opinion • Case studies • Studies of poor methodological quality	• Expert opinion • Case studies • Studies of poor methodological quality

Table 53.1   Quality appraisal of evidence.

- Is the research question valid and clearly stated?
- Is the research design and methodological approach robust and appropriate to answer the research question?
- How was the data collected and were ethical implication considered?
- How was the data analysed, are all details included so that you can identify how the researchers draw their conclusions?
- Are the results relevant and applicable to my practice?

Long-term Conditions in Adults at a Glance, First Edition. Edited by Aby Mitchell, Barry Hill, and Ian Peate.

This chapter will offer a definition of evidence-based practice, explore why it is important, how it can be generated and how nursing can critically appraise the quality of evidence they use to support their practice. Despite all the challenges of nursing today, our ability to apply evidence-based practice has been described as critical in assuring high-quality patient care.

Nurse education

The historical view of nursing has suggested that it relied on practical skills rather than intelligence and appropriated other professional language to demonstrate an understanding of education and research. However, nursing has been a graduate profession for almost a decade and throughout their undergraduate educational experience and their continuing professional development nurses are encouraged to use evidence to support their practice. The most recent update to nursing professional standards describes the need to imbed an understanding and application of research into the undergraduate programme. Yet, many nurses cite their experience as being what informs their practice and that the research process that develops evidence remains distinct from the reality of this practice.

What is evidence-based practice?

Evidence-based practice is a problem-solving approach to clinical decision-making that incorporates a search for the best and latest evidence, clinical expertise and assessment, and patient preferences and values, within a context of caring.

Rather than the evidence being distinct from practice, what constitutes evidence includes patient experience, nurses experience *and* research generated evidence.

The steps that encourage evidence-based practice include:
- identifying a question related to clinical practice
- using a systematic approach when searching for evidence
- critically appraising to assure the evidence is high quality
- using this evidence alongside nursing and patient experience and expertise to inform practice
- evaluating the impact of this on practice
- disseminating high quality evidence-based practice.

What are the perceived or actual barriers to nurses applying evidence-based practice?

The nursing profession continues to be described as lacking a robust research culture. Nurses describe the barriers to implementing evidence-based health care and these include a lack of resources, including a lack of time, lack of support from leaders and a lack of confidence in their understanding of the evidence. This seems to revert to the conclusion that nurses do not have the confidence to firstly appraise the quality of evidence, or the confidence to challenge established practice by applying new evidence to their practice.

A reliance on search engines such as GOOGLE is concerning but often nurses will also cite guidelines and policies without recognising them as secondary data. This acceptance without questioning or exploration could be attributed to a lack of time, but does not allow a critical appraisal of the primary evidence which informs the guidelines. Evidence that can be, at times, limited. Identifying what is good quality evidence is the first step of applying evidence-based practice.

Hierarchy of evidence-based practice

The quality of evidence is often presented as a pyramid – at the top are systematic reviews along with multi-centre experimental studies. Below are randomised controlled trials, observational and interpretive studies followed by non-randomised studies, descriptive studies, or action research. The lowest level of the pyramid includes expert opinion case studies and those identified as having a poor methodological approach (Figure 53.1). Nurses should aim to identify the highest level of evidence that has been generated to support their practice. This may mean using available evidence that is not at the top of the pyramid, but not that it cannot support the development high quality practice. Once you have identified the highest quality evidence available it is important to critically appraise the evidence. There are frameworks available such as Critical Appraisal Skills Programme (Table 53.1). These offer a robust structure to assure you have considered all aspects of quality assurance. The questions below are also examples of what you may consider when appraising the quality of evidence.

Knowledge translation

We have explored the barriers to nurses using evidence-based practice which includes the pressure of clinical practice, but perhaps the most important factor is the relevance to our practice. One study describes how there remains a gap between evidence and practice and nurses should employ a knowledge translation approach to bridge this gap. By working together with educational, practice and researcher partners there can be a joint construction of evidence derived from nursing and patient experience. Similarly, by encouraging nurses working in practice to co-construct formal research studies we assure their validity and impact on quality health care. This experience and expertise are how we decide whether the evidence can be applied to our practice.

54 Leadership and management

Barry Hill

Table 54.1 The nine dimensions of leadership.

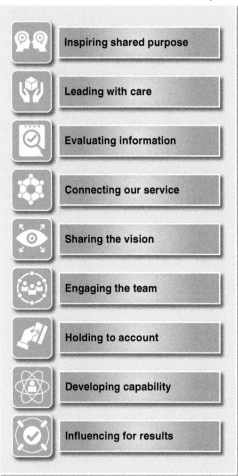

Inspiring shared purpose

Leading with care

Evaluating information

Connecting our service

Sharing the vision

Engaging the team

Holding to account

Developing capability

Influencing for results

Developing the right people with the right skills and the right values is recognised as a key priority to enable the sustainable delivery of health services, as leadership is one of the most influential factors in shaping an organisational culture. Ensuring the necessary leadership behaviours, strategies and qualities are developed is fundamental. In recent years, mandates from the government to Health Education England (HEE) and NHS England have highlighted the importance of leadership. The NHS needs high quality leaders at every level and in every area to ensure that it can deliver high quality compassionate care to the people it serves. This is more important now than ever as the health service changes to deliver new models of care.

Leaders come in many different forms and can operate at any level, so the ability to identify and develop leaders can be challenging. Yet, when done correctly, leadership can bring about positive outcomes for people, businesses, and wider communities. As the current business context is requiring organisations to become more agile, so it requires a fresh understanding of what constitutes leadership. There is an increasing recognition that all employees need to be leaders within the context of their operating level and organisational requirements. It is important to note that successful leaders do not always behave in identical ways. They may act very differently, even in similar situations, and have quite different personalities. Different leadership qualities may be needed in different circumstances.

The role of leadership in an organisation is crucial in terms of creating a vision, mission, determination, and establishment of objectives, designing strategies, policies, and methods to achieve the organisational objectives effectively and efficiently along with directing and coordinating the efforts and organisational activities. Leadership style is a combination of different characteristics, traits and behaviours that are used by leaders for interacting with their teammates. Leadership styles can be considered as a relationship that is used by an individual to make people work together for a common goal or objective.

Long-term Conditions in Adults at a Glance, First Edition. Edited by Aby Mitchell, Barry Hill, and Ian Peate.
© 2023 John Wiley & Sons Ltd. Published 2023 by John Wiley & Sons Ltd.

The NHS Leadership Academy (2014) created the nine dimensions of the health-care leadership models (Table 54.1). They note that the way that health-care professionals manage themselves is a central part of being an effective leader. It is vital to recognise that personal qualities like self-awareness, self-confidence, self-control, self-knowledge, personal reflection, resilience, and determination are the foundation of how people behave. Being aware of strengths and limitations in these areas will have a direct effect on behaviour and interaction with others. Without this awareness, it will be much more difficult to behave effectively. This, in turn, will have a direct impact on colleagues, any teamwork, and the overall culture and climate within the team as well as within the organisation. Whether health-care professionals work directly with patients and service users or not, this can affect the care experience they have. Working positively on these personal qualities will lead to a focus on care and high-quality services for patients and service users, their carer's and their families.

Some of the most common types of leadership styles are discussed below.

Autocratic style

Autocratic leadership, also known as authoritarian leadership, is a leader who has full control over distribution of workload and responsibility. An autocratic leader does not take input from other members of the team when making decisions. Operations, methods, processes, and delegation are all decided by the autocratic leader and the autocratic leader only.

Democratic style

The democratic leadership style is also called the participative style as it encourages employees to be a part of the decision-making. The democratic manager keeps his or her employees informed about everything that affects their work and shares decision-making and problem-solving responsibilities. This style requires the leader to be a coach who has the final say but gathers information from staff members before making a decision. Democratic leadership can produce high quality and high quantity work for long periods of time. Many employees like the trust they receive and respond with cooperation, team spirit, and high morale.

Laissez-faire style

The laissez-faire leadership style is also known as the 'hands-off' style. It is one in which the manager provides little or no direction and gives employees as much freedom as possible. All authority or power is given to the employees, and they must determine goals, make decisions, and resolve problems on their own.

Bureaucratic style

Bureaucratic leadership can be defined as a system of management that follows a hierarchy where official duties are fixed. Employees in this form of leadership are expected to follow specific rules and authority created by their superiors.

Situational style

Situational leadership is a style of leadership where leaders consider the readiness level of the team members they serve and the uniqueness of every situation.

Transactional style

Transactional leadership is characterised by control, organisation, and short-term planning. Leaders who adopt this style rely on a system of rewards and punishment to motivate their followers. There are also a few key assumptions associated with transactional leadership that suggest that rewards and punishments are motivating for followers of this style

Transformational style

Transformational leadership is a leadership style in which leaders encourage, inspire and motivate employees to innovate and create change that will help grow and shape the future success of the team and overall workplace.

Organisational culture

The organisational culture in which leaders and managers work has a critical bearing on their ability to do their job effectively. As well as maintaining stability at executive level, both in terms of personnel and strategic approach, many of the best performing provider organisations in the UK have focused on developing an inclusive and respectful culture and promoting good communication across the workforce. For example, the leaders and managers of these organisations are often skilled in brokering agreement between a diverse range of professionals and in ensuring that change is shaped and owned by front-line teams, rather than imposed from above and driven by a handful of senior figures. They also support initiatives aimed at breaking down inter-professional boundaries and fostering a sense of shared purpose across the organisation. The presence of an inclusive culture, as described in the NHS People Plan (NHS England 2020) geared towards learning and knowledge sharing, is critical in enabling managers to communicate well, build effective teams and establish good relationships with their senior colleagues, peers, and direct reports. The RCN (2022) identify that leaders are critical in shaping organisational culture. Nurses prefer managers who are participative, facilitative and emotionally intelligent. Leadership styles contribute to team cohesion, lower stress, and higher empowerment and self-efficacy. Leadership is a predictor of quality outcomes in health-care settings. Authentic leaders offer good role models consistent with values and vision for health care. They offer individualised consideration of staff, provide motivation, and stimulate creativity and innovation. Collective leadership is a more recent area of interest. It reflects the assumption that acts of leadership should come from anybody, not only those in formal positions of authority. Finally, there has been much investment in leadership programmes. However, the evidence base for leadership interventions remains unclear.

Chronic pain management

55

Claire Ford and Laura Park

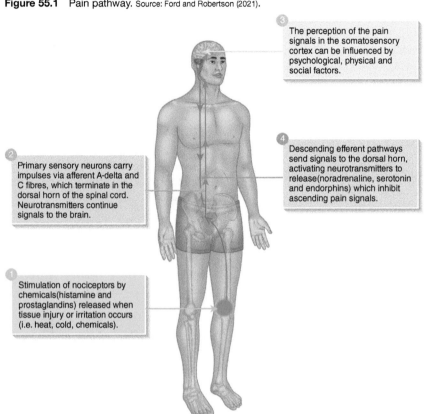

Figure 55.1   Pain pathway. Source: Ford and Robertson (2021).

3 The perception of the pain signals in the somatosensory cortex can be influenced by psychological, physical and social factors.

2 Primary sensory neurons carry impulses via afferent A-delta and C fibres, which terminate in the dorsal horn of the spinal cord. Neurotransmitters continue signals to the brain.

4 Descending efferent pathways send signals to the dorsal horn, activating neurotransmitters to release(noradrenaline, serotonin and endorphins) which inhibit ascending pain signals.

1 Stimulation of nociceptors by chemicals(histamine and prostaglandins) released when tissue injury or irritation occurs (i.e. heat, cold, chemicals).

Figure 55.2   Example of assessment domains.

Physical appearance
- Facial expressions
- Postering
- Guarding
- Reduced movement
- Abnormal gait
- Body language

Physical impact
- Bowel habits
- Insominia
- Fatigue
- Vital signs

Pain characteristics
- Location
- Duration
- Intensity
- Characteristics
- Precipitating or aggravating factors

Emotional / Behavioural
- Depression
- Anger
- Irritability
- Vocalisations

Quality of life
- Social activities
- Relationships
- Work
- Cultural impact
- Religion

Past experiences
- Coping strategies
- Medications
- Expectations

Figure 55.3   Classifications of pharmacological analgesics (examples).

Non-opioids / NSAID's
- Paracetamol
- Aspirin
- Ibuprofen
- Naproxen
- Diclofenac

Opioids
- Codeine
- Fentanyl
- Morphine
- Oxycodone
- Tramadol

Adjuvants / Co-Analgesics
- Gabapentin
- Pregabalin
- Duloxetine
- Ketamine
- Amitriptyline

Long-term Conditions in Adults at a Glance, First Edition. Edited by Aby Mitchell, Barry Hill, and Ian Peate.
© 2023 John Wiley & Sons Ltd. Published 2023 by John Wiley & Sons Ltd.

Figure 55.4 Non-pharmacology management strategies.

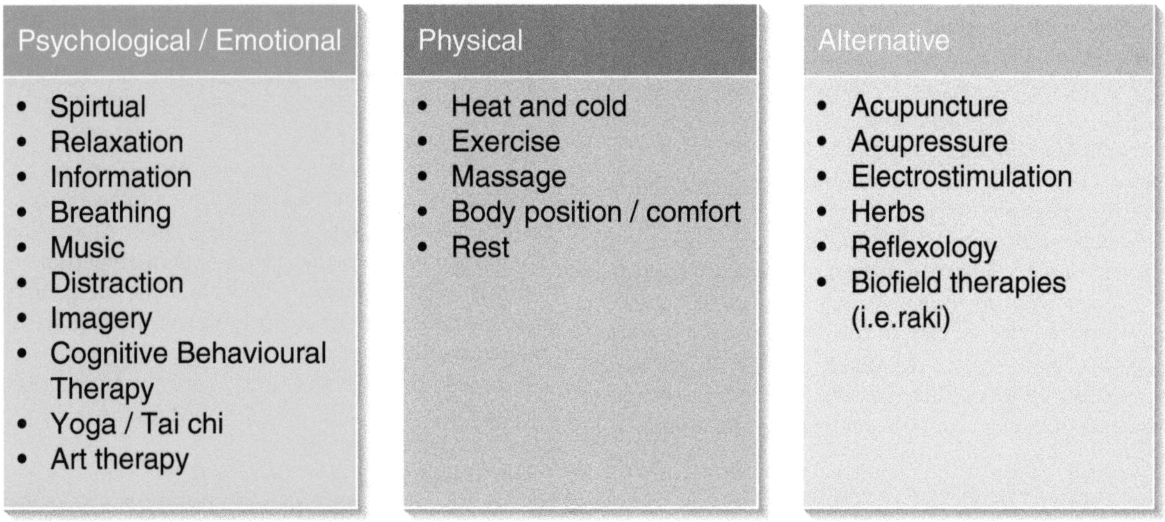

Psychological / Emotional	Physical	Alternative
• Spirtual • Relaxation • Information • Breathing • Music • Distraction • Imagery • Cognitive Behavioural Therapy • Yoga / Tai chi • Art therapy	• Heat and cold • Exercise • Massage • Body position / comfort • Rest	• Acupuncture • Acupressure • Electrostimulation • Herbs • Reflexology • Biofield therapies (i.e.raki)

Pain is usually associated with an unpleasant sensory and emotional experience associated with actual or potential tissue damage. However, pain is not always directly linked to the amount of trauma as it can also be associated with psychological and emotional issues. This is especially true regarding chronic pain, which is largely neuropathic, associated with an array of changes to the pain pathway (see Figure 55.1), and usually treated alongside psychological measures due to its extremely subjective nature. It also serves no protective purpose and is described as pain that persists or recurs for more than three months.

Globally chronic pain is one of the most prominent causes of disability and is the most common reason for someone seeking medical attention. The prevalence of chronic pain is also said to increase with age and is documented to be more prevalent amongst women and individuals who live in deprived areas, are obese, smoke, are inactive, are unemployed, or work in manual occupations.

Causes of chronic pain

There are multiple reasons why someone may develop chronic pain; however, back pain, headaches and joint pain are the most common types reported.

Other causes include:
• Injury
• Surgical intervention
• Ongoing degenerative conditions
• Fractures
• Poor posture
• Overuse/repetitive use of limbs/muscles
• Connective tissue disorders.

Chronic pain assessment

Chronic pain often detrimentally impacts people's lives as the signs and symptoms associated can extend beyond the physical sensations of burning, throbbing, aching, and shooting, with most sufferers experiencing impaired function, limits to their

daily activities and an overall reduction in quality of life. Therefore, to ensure an effective and individually tailored holistic management plan is developed, it is important to understand how the pain is uniquely affecting the individuals, from a biopsychosocial perspective. To do this, health-care professionals use a range of tools, such as the skills of observation (the art of noticing), questioning techniques, active listening and interpretation. It is important to remember that no one skill is superior, rather it is the culmination of information gathered via the various methods that enable health-care professionals to determine if a patient is in pain and more importantly understand how this pain is affecting them physically, psychologically, socially, and culturally (see Figure 55.2).

Chronic pain assessments should therefore include exploration of the following:
• **Sleep:** Reduced sleep is a common complaint as certain positions adopted in bed may cause pain to intensify and flare-ups in pain can sometimes occur at night. Sleep can also be affected by mood such as anxiety which is another sign and symptom of chronic pain.
• **Mood:** Chronic pain can lead to feelings of anxiety and depression.
• **Diet:** Chronic pain can influence diet and many patients experience a loss of appetite or find it difficult to maintain a healthy diet, due to fatigue and reduced mobility.
• **Socialisation:** Chronic pain can leave patients feeling isolated, due to reductions in social activities.
• **Sexuality:** Chronic pain can have an impact on sexual relationships, due to reduced or painful mobility and low libido levels.

Chronic pain management

To treat patients' chronic pain successfully and holistically, management plans should incorporate a multi-modal approach using a range of pharmacological and non-pharmacological strategies. The individual should also be included in the management discussion and decision, so an understanding can be gained of personalised goals and priorities.

Pharmacological strategies

Analgesia can be categorised as opioids, which can be strong (morphine) or weak (codeine), non-opioids/non-steroidal anti-inflammatories (NSAIDs), and adjuvants/co-analgesics (see Figure 55.3). The most efficient pharmacological regimen for chronic pain often incorporates a combined approach, by administrating a specific drug in conjunction with adjuvants or co-analgesics, as several drugs have morphine-sparing properties and can also promote sleep and psychological symptoms. Gabapentinoids, such as pregabalin and gabapentin are one of the most widely used adjuvant/co-analgesic for neuropathic pain. These were developed to mimic the neurotransmitter GABA; however, while they do not bind to the GABA receptors in the central nervous system, they do inhibit calcium channels by reducing the number of available channels. This in turn prevents the neuropathic pain response from continuing to the brain.

Non-pharmacological strategies

Pharmacological treatments are not the only strategy at health-care professionals' disposal, and true holistic management cannot be achieved without the incorporation of other non-pharmacological therapies, which when used correctly, may reduce some of the debilitating symptoms and can enhance sleep and overall well-being. These treatments can be placed into three main groups (see Figure 55.4) and the choice of which to use will depend upon patients' preferences and existing coping mechanisms.

- **Distraction:** This can take various forms, i.e. talking to the patient about their specific hobbies. This basic skill often requires no equipment, can be done anywhere, and is a useful way of taking the patient's mind off their pain.
- **Imagery/meditation:** This management technique takes distraction therapy one step further by utilising a more structured approach.
- **Therapeutic touch and massage:** For centuries, the therapeutic placing of hands has proven to be a useful skill and has beneficial physiological (stimulation of A-beta fibres which restrict pain pathways) and psychological properties.
- **Environment:** Sound, lighting and the temperature of the patient's immediate environment has been shown to heighten or reduce perceptions of pain.
- **Acupuncture:** This technique is often used as a management approach for chronic pain as it stimulates the natural release of pain-relieving endorphins.
- **Cognitive behavioural therapy (CBT):** This is a psychological approach to managing pain, which looks to address an individual's emotional experience to pain so that it can be self-managed.
- **Exercise:** Exercise such as yoga, swimming and walking are encouraged, as they have been shown to reduce pain and stiffness. Physiotherapy can also be recommended to not only relieve pain but also as a useful tool to find alternative ways to engage with daily activities. However, physiotherapy and exercise should be prescribed with caution, to reduce the risk of causing further strain or injury.

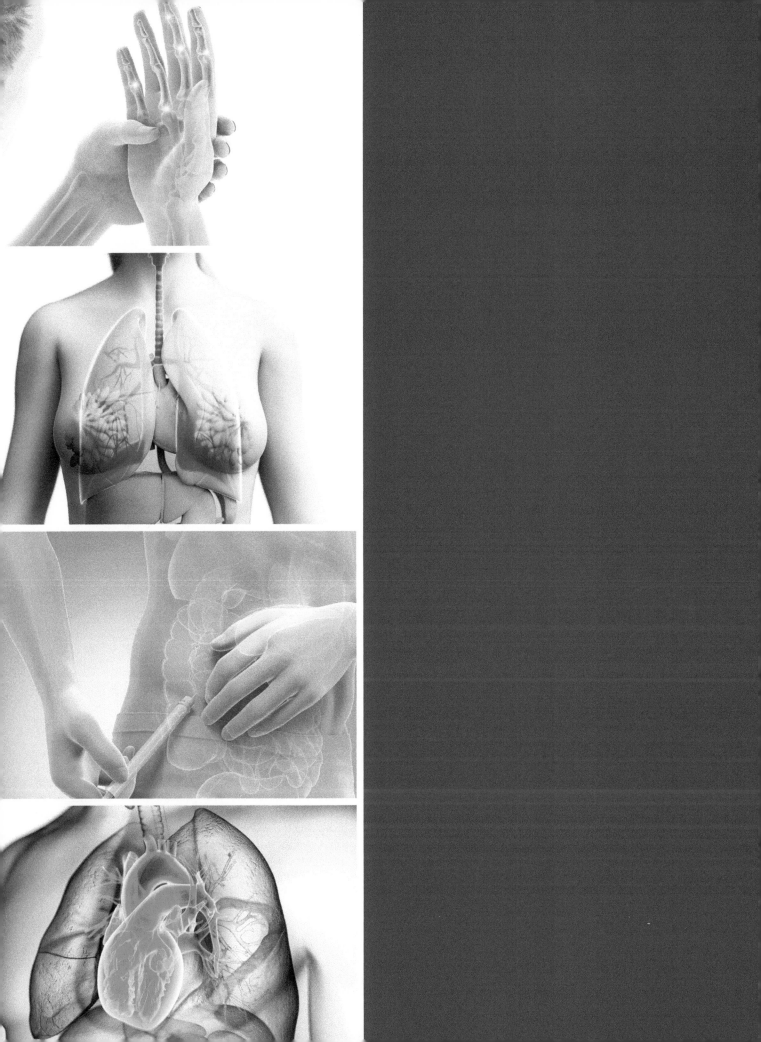

56

56 End of life care

Jemma-Louise McCann and Sara Sinclair

Table 56.1 Some therapeutic medications used in EoLC.

Drugs	Indications	Contraindications	Common starting doses for continuous subcutaneous infusion (CSI) or PRN (guide only, specialist palliative care staff may recommend outside usual range)
Pain			
Morphine sulphate (10 mg/1 ml ampules)	Pain or breathlessness First line analgesia	Poor kidney function/ allergies to morphine sulphate or hallucinations	CSI: 5–10 mg/24 hr if no current opioid usage PRN: 2.5–5 mg/hourly (pain) 1.25–2.5 mg/hourly (breathlessness)
Oxycodone (10 mg/1 ml ampules)	Pain or breathlessness Second line if morphine not indicated	Allergies	CSI: 2.5–5 mg/24 hr PRN: 1.25–2.5 mg/hourly (pain or breathlessness)
Anti-emetics			
Levomepromazine (25 mg/1 ml ampules)	Nausea, vomiting or terminal agitation (Second line to midazolam for agitation)	Allergies Parkinson's disease	CSI: 6.25–25 mg/24 hr PRN: 6.25 mg/12 hr (for antiemetic) 6.25 mg/4 hr for agitation
Sedative			
Midazolam (10 mg/2 ml)	Terminal agitation or seizures	Allergies	CSI: 5–15 mg/24 hr for Agitation if no prior usage 20–30 mg/24 hr for convulsions (or risk of convulsions) PRN: 2.5–5 mg/2 hr 10 mg stat repeat after 15 min for catastrophic bleeds or convulsions
Anticholinergics			
Hyoscine butylbromide (20 mg/1 ml)	Chest secretions/bowel obstruction (First line)	Allergies	CSI: 40–120 mg/24 hr for chest secretions 60–300 mg/24 hr for bowel obstruction PRN: 20 mg/4 hr

One chance to get it right

The leading causes of death in the UK in 2018 was ischaemic heart disease, specifically linked with congestive heart failure and strokes, closely followed by dementia and Alzheimer's disease. Many of these conditions can be linked to societies ageing population and subsequent co-morbidities. Through disease progression patients will require palliative care support. Palliative care is defined as emotional, practical and physical, support to people with a terminal illness and can be offered at any point after diagnosis. However, palliative care and end-of-life care are terms that are often used interchangeably. Palliative care can often be measured on a trajectory; however, there is only a diagnosis of end-of-life when the patient is in the last 6–12 months of life and end-of-life care involves those patients being able to obtain appropriate treatment, care and support.

Indicators of end-of-life care include

- Progressive incurable aggressive cancers.
- Advanced disease progression within long-term conditions.
- Extensive frailty.
- Catastrophic events leading to life-threatening conditions.

End-of-life care is multi-faceted and includes supporting patients through, emotional, physical, spiritual, and social aspects of their care.

The Gold Standards Framework

The End-of-Life Care (EoLC) strategy reports that when services are commissioned provisions for EoLC, they are required to follow a systematic and evidence-based approach, utilising quality assured tools for effective management. One of these quality assured tools is the Gold Standards Framework (GSF). The GSF aims to improve palliative care and end-of-life care provided by health and social-care professionals in the community, by actively identifying or 'caseload finding' individuals who might be nearing the end of life. Once an individual is identified, the health and social-care team can undertake a holistic assessment to support a plan of care. The GSF focuses on enabling continuity of care, teamwork, advanced planning, symptom control and patient support which is inclusive of their carer's and family. The GSF guides health professionals with prompts and tools to help them identify when someone may be entering the end-of-life phase of their illness, i.e. the last 6–12 months of their lives.

Long-term Conditions in Adults at a Glance, First Edition. Edited by Aby Mitchell, Barry Hill, and Ian Peate.
© 2023 John Wiley & Sons Ltd. Published 2023 by John Wiley & Sons Ltd.

Symptoms of end-of-life

- Extreme fatigue.
- Reduced abilities to self-manage and increased use of support services for activities of daily living.
- Reduced or limited mobility often resulting in bed-bound status.
- Delirium or confusion and or increased agitation.
- Loss of mechanical functions of swallowing therefore, reduced oral intake (food and drink) and difficulty swallowing medication.
- Reduction in efficient blood circulation, resulting in the body conserving heat centrally (resulting in cold extremities).
- Inability to control continence functions, either loss of control or ability to expel.
- Conversing with others becomes difficult and non-existent.
- Changes in breathing can result in breathlessness.

Actively dying phase

The time in which a person is actively dying is denoted as the last 48 hours of life and often at this stage, patients exhibit some of the following symptoms:

- Agitation and restlessness: often misconstrued as pain or convulsions. May include waving arms, kicking of the legs, aimlessly plucking, moaning and visual distress.
- Secretions from the upper airways: caused by deterioration in swallowing and patient unable to clear fluid from airways. This is referred to as the 'death rattle' (often more distressing for witnesses than the patient).
- Pain: this can be expressed verbally or non-verbally, such as facial expressions, groans and lashing out.
- Vomiting and nausea: common at end-of-life, likely causes include hypercalcaemia, bowel obstructions, renal cancers, and side-effects from analgesia.

Continuous subcutaneous infusions

Medications commonly used to control these symptoms can be found in Table 56.1. This list not exhaustive; it is only an example and should be only used in conjunction with the prescribing practitioner's assessment. All prescribers and nurses administering medication are required to be aware of the medication compatibilities and adhere to local policies. All these symptoms need to be anticipated and proactively planned to prevent a crisis. Patients who are diagnosed as end-of-life can move into the active stage of dying rapidly and therefore, when effectively planning for EoLC, anticipatory medication (known as Just in Case drugs) should be in place ready to use if needed. Injections are often used in the latter stages of EoLC for reasons such as: the inability to swallow medications, there is uncontrolled nausea or vomiting, uncontrolled escalating pain and or agitation and absorption issues. A continuous subcutaneous infusion should be started via a delivery pump often known as a syringe pump.

Implantable cardioverter defibrillators (ICDs)/pacemakers

Implantable cardioverter defibrillators (ICD)/pacemakers are devices that support the function of the heart. Pacemakers work from the electrical activity of the heart; they do not need to be turned off at end-of-life. However, ICDs send electrical shocks to restart the heart; therefore, at end-of-life they will need to be turned off and discussion should form part of the advanced care planning.

Other considerations include

- Culture differences, religious ceremonies, and spiritual needs of individuals at end-of-life.
- Oxygen therapy to be reviewed if required as essential.
- Mouth care should be performed to support patient comfort.
    More information can be found at: www.mariecurie.org.uk; 'One chance to get it right' GOV.UK, 2015.

DEATH: after care and support

- Verification of death.
- Contact NOK/relatives.
- Contact any religious leaders and/or hospital chaplaincy.
- Removal of foreign bodies, i.e. catheters, cannulas, syringe pump.
- Perform last offices (known as the respectful process of caring for the body after death).

Bereavement

Bereavement is the process of mourning the loss of a relationship and can affect anyone in contact with the deceased. This process can cause both physical and emotional responses.

    Support groups and counselling services for bereavement: www.mind.org.uk; Cruise Bereavement Care 0808 808 1677.

57 Advanced care planning

Sara Sinclair

Table 57.1 The six steps approach when considering ACP.

1. Identify: Patient-centred care plan to suit their own requests and needs.
2. Assess: Personalised focus on things that matter to the patient.
3. Discuss: Consent from the patient is essential.
4. Plan: Sharing the Advanced Care Plan.
5. Coordinate: All individuals involved must be given the opportunity to review, adapt and change the Advanced Care Plan.
6. Review: Everyone involved must be able to be open and honest throughout the process.

Table 57.2 The patient's understanding of key information.

- Capacity and consent from the patient are essential when developing an ACP.
- Information regarding their own health, condition and prognosis.
- The processes involved in advanced care planning.
- Aspects of care to consider.
- How can these be altered or changed?
- Can any amendment be made and what is the process?
- How can I nominate an advocate to make decisions if I am unable to make these decisions?
- Who can support me through the process?

Table 57.3 The most commonly identified circumstances where ACP are not implemented (National Institute for Health and Care Excellence 2019).

- Medical emergencies, i.e. car crash, unexpected pulmonary infarction etc.
- Dementia patients – often patients are not diagnosed until the later stages of the disease process and therefore, unfortunately maybe unable to make informed decisions at the time of formal diagnosis.
- Patient decline to make ACP or are suffering denial of their disease, condition and prognosis.
- Patients are scared to involve or tell family of their conditions or do not want to burden their family with their needs, preferences, and concerns.

Long-term Conditions in Adults at a Glance, First Edition. Edited by Aby Mitchell, Barry Hill, and Ian Peate.
© 2023 John Wiley & Sons Ltd. Published 2023 by John Wiley & Sons Ltd.

Advanced care planning (ACP) is defined as a voluntary process of understanding an individual's personal preferences, goals and values. The aim is to impart their own visions prior to an individual becoming end-of-life, critically unwell or being unable to make informed decisions. This is intended to enable individuals with life-limiting conditions or serious illness to receive medical treatment and care in line with their own personal needs, values and preferences. The National Institute for Health and Care Excellence (2022) report ACP can consist of different approaches: advanced statements, Lasting Power of Attorney (LPA) and advanced decisions.

Advanced statement: Refers to written or verbal information regarding aspects a person considers important to their health and well-being. These are not legal documents and may not always be able to be followed. However, when planning care in practice health-care professionals (HCPs) will consider aspects of the advanced statement.

LPA: The document a person uses when nominating or, legally giving consent for a trusted individual to make informed decisions: when they are unable to make their own informed decisions regarding health and welfare and/or property and financial affairs. Medical decisions can only be made if a LPA is for Health and Welfare. All LPA must be registered with the Office of the Public Guardian and is only effective at the point the person is deemed not to have capacity.

Advanced decision to refuse treatment

Advanced Decision to Refuse Treatment (ADRT) provides an individual with the tools to implement measures to identify their own preference to decline treatment independently of the likely outcome or procedure. ADRT allows a person to make choices to refuse ventilation, PEG feeding and other treatments. These decisions are known as 'life sustaining' or 'life prolonging decisions'. It is important to recognise ADRT are unable to be implemented to make a request to end one's life or to decline basic human rights such as keeping safe, access to nutrition and hydration, and being comfortable and warm. Discussions around ADRT are usually carried out in consultation with a person's general practitioner (GP) or appropriate health-care professional (HCPs). An ADRT needs to be specific itemising the the treatment being refused. It must be written down, witnessed and signed following the correct legal measures to be a legally binding directive.

ReSPECT document

In more recent years some localities have implemented the Recommended Summary Plan for Emergency Care and Treatment (ReSPECT) forms are clinical guidance stating the persons wishes in an emergency situation, when they unable to make decisions about their care/ health. It is recommended that these conversations take place between the patient, family and HCPs as a shared decision. Further information on the ReSPECT document can be found from the Resuscitation Council UK (2020). The Department of Health and Social Care (DHSC) sets out a six-step approach when considering ACP (Table 57.1).

Implementing/developing an ACP/ADRT/ReSPECT plan

It is important to consider that not everyone will want an advanced care plan in place. Implementing an ACP can be

a sensitive subject for many people. Therefore, caution and care should be taken when introducing the idea of ceilings of care especially in patients with recent diagnoses or a notification of prognosis. However, should a person decide to create an ACP there is a series of aspects to be considered. Most importantly it is essential for mental capacity to be assessed by an appropriately trained HCP. When assessing capacity, the HCP should ensure the person has the ability to make a decision and be able to understand the implications and consequences of that decision. It is essential mental capacity is assessed to ensure the person is able to understand the information regarding their health, care and future. The person must be able to retain the information provided and show evidence that they are able to weigh up the pros and cons of the decision (The Mental Capacity Act 2005).

The difference between ReSPECT and DNACPR

Do not attempt cardiopulmonary resuscitation (DNACPR) decisions is a document that authorises HCPs to not attempt CPR: if a person's heart stopped pumping. DNACPR only discusses CPR options without any variation in circumstance. However, the ReSPECT form evidences the persons preferences and wishes in an emergency situation. It may include decisions around DNRCPR. CPR is a procedure used in emergencies to attempt to get the heart re-beating and to get oxygen around the body to vital organs. However, it can cause other serious life-limiting complications. There are several factors the patient must be aware of when the ReSPECT form is considered (NHS England 2018) (Table 57.2).

Creating the ACP/ADRT/ReSPECT

Once the patient has considered all their needs and preferences, it is important to discuss these with the HCPs to create a document. All the information regarding their preferences, decisions and plans need to be written clearly and signed by the HCP (with authority to do so). The patient/carer/family can sign the ReSPECT form however, this is not essential.

What happens if there is not an ACP/ADRT/ReSPECT in place?

If a person has not considered or documented their preferences before suffering a life-threatening emergency, or conditions which prevent them from being able to make an informed decision, the HCPs will make appropriate clinical decisions in the best interests of the patient, following a mental capacity assessment under the Mental Capacity Act (2005). When making in best interest decisions those who know the person best should ideally be involved in the process.

ACP's which are in place are not always implemented. This can be attributed to several factors (Table 57.3) including non adherence by health professionals or inaccuracies in the ACP such as inaccessibility of the plans, plans providing ambiguous or conflicting instructions, and inappropriate focus on the completion of documents rather than communication.

Advanced care planning is an important aspect of care intended to enable individuals to receive medical treatment at the end of life in line with their own beliefs, values and wishes. Healthcare professionals must be aware of patients wishes to help prioritise future care.

Bibliography

Chapter 1

Dahlgren, G. and Whitehead, M. (1991). *Policies and Strategies to Promote Social Equity in Health*. Stockholm: Institute for Futures Studies.

Dahlgren, G. and Whitehead, M. (2021). The Dahlgren-Whitehead model of health determinants: 30 years on and still chasing rainbows. *Public Health* 199: 20–24.

Department of Health and Social Care (2023). Care and support statutory guidance. https://www.gov.uk/government/publications/care-act-statutory-guidance/care-and-support-statutory-guidance (accessed 27 March 2023).

Kane, R. and Reilly, R. (2011). Tackling health inequalities. In: *Nursing for Public Health: Promotion, Principles and Practice* (ed. P. Linsley, R. Kane, and S. Owen), 175–189. Oxford: Oxford University Press.

National Health Service (2019). The NHS long term plan. National Health Service. https://www.longtermplan.nhs.uk/wp-content/uploads/2019/08/nhs-long-term-plan-version-1.2.pdf (accessed 17 May 2022).

Chapter 2

Public Health England (2017). Research and analysis. Chapter 5: inequality in health. http://www.gov.uk/government/publications/health-profile-for-england/chapter-5-inequality-in-health (accessed 22 April 2022).

Royal College of Nursing (2012). *Health Inequalities and the Social Determinants of Health*. London: RCN.

Williams, E., Buck, D., and Babalola, G. (2020). What are health inequalities. www.kingsfund.org.uk/publications/what-are-health-inequalities#what (accessed 22 April 2022).

Chapter 3

Department of Health/Long-term Conditions (2012). Long-term conditions compendium of Information: 3rd edition. https://assets.publishing.service.gov.uk/government/uploads/system/uploads/attachment_data/file/216528/dh_134486.pdf (accessed 15 May 2022).

Environment Agency (2021). State of the environment: health, people and the environment. https://www.gov.uk/government/publications/state-of-the-environment/state-of-the-environment-health-people-and-the-environment#fn:7 (accessed 12 April 2022).

Sly, P.D., Carpenter, D.O., Van den Berg, M. et al. (2016). Health consequences of environmental exposures: causal thinking in global environmental epidemiology. *Ann. Glob. Health* 82 (1): 3–9. https://doi.org/10.1016/j.aogh.2016.01.004 (accessed 12 April 2022).

Chapter 4

Mind (2014). Mind guide to housing and mental health. www.mindcharity.co.uk/wp-content/uploads/2013/05/guide-to-housing_2014.pdf (accessed 22 April 2022).

Public Health England (2017). Homes for older people. Housing infographics slides updated with disclaimer slide.pptx. Powered by Box.

Shelter (2017). The impact of housing problems on mental health. https://assets.ctfassets.net/6sxvmndnpn0s/59MBno13nAzVDGZeSjiJkX/3c2b8e75becb0e3f10057f696c95c284/Housing_and_mental_health_-_detailed_report.pdf (accessed 22 April 2022).

Chapter 5

National Institute for Health and Care Excellence (2020). Behaviour change: digital and mobile health interventions. www.nice.org.uk/guidance/ng183/resources/behaviour-change-digital-and-mobile-health-interventions-pdf-66142020002245 (accessed 22 April 2022).

Public Health England and Health Education England (2018). Making every contact count (MECC): implementation guide. MECC Implementation Guide. http://publishing.service.gov.uk (accessed 22 March 2022).

Public Health England (2021). All our health: personalised care and population health. http://www.gov.uk/government/collections/all-our-health-personalised-care-and-population-health (accessed 22 April 2022).

Chapter 6

Davey, P., Rathmell, A., Dunn, M. et al. (2017). *Medical Ethics, Law and Communication at a Glance*. Oxford: Wiley.

Prochaska, J.O. and DiClemente, C.C. (1983). Stages and processes of self change of smoking: towards an integrative module of change. *J. Consult. Clin. Psychol.* 51 (1): 390–395.

Royal College of Nursing (2019). Understanding behaviour change. www.rcn.org.uk/clinical-topics/supporting-behaviour-change/understanding-behaviour-change (accessed 22 April 2022).

Chapter 7

Barnett, K., Mercer, S.W., Norbury, M. et al. (2012). Epidemiology of multimorbidity and implications for health care, research, and medical education: a cross-sectional study. *Lancet* 380 (9836): 37–43. https://doi.org/10.1016/S0140-6736(12)60240-2.

King's Fund (n.d.) Long-term conditions and multi-morbidity. www.kingsfund.org.uk/projects/time-think-differently/trends-disease-and-disability-long-term-conditions-multi-morbidity (accessed 22 April 2022).

Mair, F.S. and Jani, B.D. (2020). Emerging trends and future research on the role of socioeconomic status in chronic illness and multimorbidity. *Lancet* 5 (3): E128–E129. https://doi.org/10.1016/S2468-2667(20)30001-3.

Race Equality Foundation (2021). Long term conditions briefing paper. www.raceequalityfoundation.org.uk/wp-content/uploads/2020/06/Collaborative-briefing-long-term-health-briefing-digital-FINAL.pdf (accessed 22 April 2022).

Chapter 8

Bradbury, M. (2022). *District Nursing At a Glance*. Oxford: Wiley.

NHS (2019). The NHS long term plan. http://www.longtermplan. nhs.uk/wp-content/uploads/2019/08/nhs-long-term-plan-version-1.2.pdf (accessed 22 April 2022).

Which (2021). Getting a needs assessment. www.which.co.uk/ reviews/later-life-care/article/later-life-care/getting-a-needs-assessment-aAxfc4G7iYTt (accessed 22 April 2022).

Chapter 9

NICE (2011). Making every contact count: implementing NICE behaviour change guidance. www.nice.org.uk/sharedlearning/ making-every-contact-count-implementing-nice-behaviour-change-guidance (accessed 20 November 2020).

PHE (2016). Making every contact count (MECC) https://assets. publishing.service.gov.uk/government/uploads/system/ uploads/attachment_data/file/769486/Making_Every_Contact_ Count_Consensus_Statement.pdf (accessed 20 November 2022).

RCN (2022). Supporting behaviour change. www.rcn.org.uk/clinical-topics/supporting-behaviour-change (accessed 20 November 2022).

Chapter 10

The National Society for Marketing Centre (2022). The National Society for Marketing Behaviour. Online. Available at: https:// www.thensmc.com/what-social-marketing.

Whitehead, D. (2018). Exploring health promotion and health education in nursing. *Nurs. Stand.* 33 (8).

Wills, J. (2014). *Fundamentals of Health Promotion for Nurses*, 2e. Oxford: Wiley.

Chapter 11

Department of Health and Social Care (2021). The NHS Constitution for England. http://www.gov.uk/government/publications/the-nhs-constitution-for-england/the-nhs-constitution-for-england (accessed 22 April 2022).

Department of Health and Social Care (2022). Handbook to the NHS Constitution for England. http://www.gov.uk/government/ publications/supplements-to-the-nhs-constitution-for-england/the-handbook-to-the-nhs-constitution-for-england (accessed 22 April 2022).

Ham, C., Charles, A., and Wellings, D. (2018). Shared responsibility for health: the cultural change we need. www.kingsfund.org.uk/ publications/shared-responsibility-health (accessed 22 April 2022).

Chapter 12

NHS England (2022). Supported self-management. https://www. england.nhs.uk/personalisedcare/supported-self-management (accessed 20 November 2022).

RCN (2022). Self-care. www.rcn.org.uk/clinical-topics/Public-health/Self-care (accessed 20 November 2022).

The Health Foundation (2022). A practical guide to self-management support: key components for successful implementation. www. health.org.uk/publications/a-practical-guide-to-self-management-support (accessed 20 November 2022).

Chapter 13

Carers UK (2022). Why we're here. www.carersuk.org (accessed 22 May 2022).

Office of National Statistics (2017). Suicide among carers and home carers in England www.ons.gov.uk/peoplepopulationand community/birthsdeathsandmarriages/deaths/adhocs/008974s uicidesamongcarersandhomecarersinengland2001to2017 (accessed 22 May 2022).

Chapter 14

Fotoukian, Z., Shahboulaghi, F.M., Khoshknab, M.F. et al. (2014). Concept analysis of empowerment in old people with chronic diseases using a hybrid model. *Asian Nurs. Res.* 8 (2): 118–127. https://doi.org/10.1016/j.anr.2014.04.002.

National Institute for Health and Care Excellence NICE (2020). Guidance on prescribing. https://bnf.nice.org.uk/guidance/ guidance-on-prescribing.html (accessed 29 March 2022).

World Health Organization (WHO) (2020). A European policy framework supporting action across government and society for health and well-being. https://www.euro.who.int/__data/assets/ pdf_file/0006/199536/Health2020-Short.pdf (accessed 29 March 2022).

Chapter 15

NHS England (2018). Personalised care operating model. https:// www.england.nhs.uk/publication/personalised-care-operating-model (accessed 20 November 2022).

NHS England (2021). Person centred care. https://www.england. nhs.uk/ourwork/patient-participation (accessed 20 November 2022).

NHS UK (2019). The NHS long term plan. https://www.long termplan.nhs.uk/publication/nhs-long-term-plan (accessed 20 November 2022).

The Kings Fund (2011). Making shared decision-making a reality: no decision about me, without me. www.kingsfund.org.uk/ publications/making-shared-decision-making-reality (accessed 20 November 2022).

Chapter 16

Gov UK (2022). Alcohol Bulletin commentary (February to April 2022). (accessed 26 June 2022).

NICE (2019). 2019 surveillance of alcohol-use disorders (NICE guidelines PH24 and CG115). https://www.nice.org.uk/guidance/ cg115/resources/2019-surveillance-of-alcoholuse-disorders-nice-guidelines-ph24-and-cg115-pdf-8866526536645 (accessed 27 March 2023).

PHE (2017). *Better Care for People with Co-Occurring Mental Health and Alcohol/Drug Use Conditions: A Guide for Commissioners and Service Providers*. London: Public Health England.

Chapter 17

National Institute for Health and Care Excellence (2017). *Eating Disorders: Recognition and Treatment*. London: NICE.

Scottish Intercollegiate Guidelines Network (SIGN) (2022). *A National Clinical Guideline on Eating Disorders*. Edinburgh: SIGN.

World Health Organisation (1992). *The ICD-10 Classification of Mental and Behavioural Disorders: Clinical Descriptions and Diagnostic Guidelines*. Geneva: WHO.

Chapter 18

National Health Service (2018). Arthritis. https://www.nhs.uk/ conditions/arthritis (accessed 22 May 2022).

National Institute for Health and Care Excellence (NICE) (2018). Rheumatoid arthritis in adults: management. [NG100] www. nice.org.uk/guidance/ng100 (accessed 22 May 2022).

National Institute for Health and Care Excellence (NICE) (2020). Osteoarthritis: care and management. [CG177] www.nice.org. uk/guidance/cg177 (accessed 22 May 2022).

Chapter 19

Asthma UK (2022). What is asthma? www.asthma.org.uk/advice/understanding-asthma/what-is-asthma (accessed 20 November 2022).

BTS and SIGN (2019). British guideline on the management of asthma (SIGN 158). British Thoracic Society and Scottish Intercollegiate Guidelines Network. https://www.brit-thoracic.org.uk (accessed 20 November 2022).

Peate, I. (ed.) (2017) *Fundamentals of Applied Pathophysiology*, 4th ed, p. 339. Oxford: Wiley-Blackwell.

WHO (2022). Asthma. https://www.who.int/news-room/fact-sheets/detail/asthma (accessed 20 November 2022).

Chapter 20

National Institute for Clinical Excellence (2011). Stable angina: management. Clinical guidelines (CG126) www.nice.org.uk/guidance/cg126 (accessed 20 November 2022).

Chapter 21

Lingwood, L., Stephenson, E., and Stavert, L. (2022). Chapter 15. In: *Fundamentals of Pharmacology for Children's Nurses* (ed. I. Peate and P. Dryden). Oxford: Wiley Blackwell.

National Institute for Health and Care Excellence (NICE) (2011). *Common Mental Health Disorders: Identification and Pathways to Care* NICE [clinical guideline: 123]. British Psychological Society and Royal College of Psychiatrists.

National Institute for Health and Care Excellence (NICE) (2014). *Anxiety Disorders Quality Standards [QS53]*. British Psychological Society and Royal College of Psychiatrists.

Chapter 22

NICE (2021). Arial fibrillation: diagnosis and management. Guideline (NG196) www.nice.org.uk/guidance/ng196 (accessed 20 November 2022).

Chapter 23

Jauhar, S., McKenna, P., and Laws, K. (2016). NICE guidance on psychological treatments for bipolar disorder: searching for the evidence. *Lancet Psychiatry* 3 (4): 386–388.

McIntyre, R., Berk, M., Brietzke, E. et al. (2020). Bipolar disorders. *Lancet* 396 (10265): 1841–1856.

Rethink Mental Illness (2022). Bipolar disorder. What are the signs and symptoms of bipolar disorder? rethink.org (accessed 17 June 2022).

Chapter 24

Kirkpatrick, J.R. (2018). *Taking a Detailed Eating Disorder History: A Comprehensive Guide for Clinicians*, 1e. New York, NY: Routledge https://doi.org/10.4324/9781315210957.

National Institute for Health and Care Excellence (NICE) (2017). *Eating Disorders: Recognition and Treatment*. London: NICE.

Scottish Intercollegiate Guidelines Network (SIGN) (2022). *A National Clinical Guideline on Eating Disorders*. Edinburgh: SIGN.

Chapter 25

Maselli, D.J., Amalakuhan, B., Keyt, H., and Diaz, A.A. (2017). Suspecting non-cystic fibrosis bronchiectasis: What the busy primary care clinician needs to know. *Int. J. Clin. Pract.* 71: e12924. https://doi.org/10.1111/ijcp.12924.

NHS (2022). Bronchiectasis. https://www.nhs.uk/conditions/bronchiectasis (accessed 20 November 2022).

NICE (2022). When should I suspect bronchiectasis? https://cks.nice.org.uk/topics/bronchiectasis/diagnosis/diagnosis (accessed 20 November 2022).

PHE (2019). UK standards for microbiology investigations. https://assets.publishing.service.gov.uk/government/uploads/system/uploads/attachment_data/file/800451/B_57i3.5.pdf (accessed 20 November 2022).

Chapter 26

Macmillan Cancer Support (2015a) Cancer in the context of other long-term conditions. Scoping evidence review and secondary data analysis. www.macmillan.org.uk/documents/press/cancerandotherlong-termconditions.pdf (accessed 20 November 2022).

Macmillan Cancer Support (2015b) The burden of cancer and other long-term health conditions. www.macmillan.org.uk/documents/press/cancerandotherlong-termconditions.pdf (accessed 20 November 2022).

McConnell, H. White, R. and Maher, J. (2015). Explaining the different complexity, intensity and longevity of broad clinical needs. www.macmillan.org.uk/_images/three-cancer-groups_tcm9-297577.pdf (accessed 22 June 2022).

Chapter 27

Bansal, R., Gubbi, S., and Koch, C.A. (2022). COVID-19 and chronic fatigue syndrome: an endocrine perspective. *J. Clin. Transl. Endocrinol.* 27: 100284. http://dx.doi.org/10.1016/j.jcte.2021.100284.

Cortes Rivera, M., Mastronardi, C., Silva-Aldana, C.T. et al. (2019). Myalgic encephalomyelitis/chronic fatigue syndrome: a comprehensive review. *Diagnostics* 9 (3): 91. https://doi.org/10.3390/diagnostics9030091.

National Institute for Health and Care Excellence (2021). Myalgic encephalomyelitis (or encephalopathy)/chronic fatigue syndrome: diagnosis and management www.nice.org.uk/guidance/ng206/chapter/Recommendations#diagnosisCEguidelines (accessed 20 November 2022).

Sapra, A. and Bhandari, P. (2022). Chronic Fatigue Syndrome. In: *StatPearls*. Treasure Island (FL): StatPearls Publishing https://www.ncbi.nlm.nih.gov/books/NBK557676.

Chapter 28

Lurie, F., Passman, M., Meisner, M. et al. (2020). The 2020 update of the CEAP classification system and reporting standards. *J. Vasc. Surg. Venous Lymphat. Disord.* 8 (3): 342–352. doi: 10.1016/j.jvsv.2019.12.075.

National Institute for Health and Care Excellence (NICE) (2021). Leg ulcer – venous. https://cks.nice.org.uk/topics/leg-ulcer-venous (accessed 6 January 2022).

Peate, I. (2021). *Fundamentals of Applied Pathophysiology*, Wiley.

Shammeri, O., AlHamdan, N., Al-hothaly, B. et al. (2014). Chronic venous insufficiency: prevalence and effect of compression stockings. Internat. *J. Health Sci.* 8 (3): 231–236.

White, J.V. and Ryjewski, C. (2005). Chronic venous insufficiency. *Perspect. Vasc. Surg. Endovasc. Ther.* 17: 319–327.

Chapter 29

Global Initiative for Chronic Obstructive Lung Disease (GOLD) (2022). Global strategy for the diagnosis, management, and prevention of chronic obstructive pulmonary disease: 2022 report. https://goldcopd.org/# (accessed 20 November 2022).

NICE (2021). Diagnosis of chronic obstructive pulmonary disease. https://cks.nice.org.uk/topics/chronic-obstructive-pulmonary-disease/diagnosis/diagnosis-copd (accessed 15 January 2022).

Chapter 30

Aaronson, P.I., Ward, J.P.T., and Connolly, M.I. (2012). *Cardiovascular System at a Glance*. Wiley, p. 76.

England, T. and Nasin, A. (2014). *ABC of Arterial and Venous Disease: ABC of Arterial and Venous Disease*. Oxford: Wiley.

National Institute of Health and Care Excellence (NICE) (2022). Acute coronary syndromes NICE guideline [NG185]. www.nice.org.uk/guidance/NG185 (accessed 22 September 2022).

National Institute of Health and Care Excellence (NICE) (2022). CVS presentation. CVD risk assessment and treatment. How NICE resources can support local priorities CVD prevention: CVD risk assessment and treatment (http://nice.org.uk) (accessed 22 September 2022).

Chapter 31

Bauersachs, R., Zeymer, U., Brière, J.B. et al. (2019). Burden of coronary artery disease and peripheral artery disease: a literature review. *Cardiovasc. Ther.* 2019: 8295054.

Joshi, D., Keane, G., Brind, A. et al. (2015). *Hepatology at a Glance*. Wiley, p. 14.

Libby, P., Ridker, P.M., and Hansson, G.K. (2011). Progress and challenges in translating the biology of atherosclerosis. *Nature* 19, 473 (7347): 317–325. https://doi.org/10.1038/nature10146. PMID: 21593864.

Shahjehan, R.D. and Bhutta, B.S. (2022). Coronary artery disease. In: *StatPearls*. Treasure Island (FL): StatPearls Publishing.

Chapter 32

British Liver Trust (2021). Statistics: liver disease crisis. https://britishlivertrust.org.uk/about-us/media-centre/statistics (accessed 20 November 2022).

Office for National Statistics (2021). Dataset: alcohol-specific deaths in the UK: liver diseases and the impact of deprivation. www.ons.gov.uk/peoplepopulationandcommunity/healthandsocialcare/causesofdeath/datasets/alcoholspecificdeathsintheunitedkingdomsupplementarydatatables (accessed 20 November 2022).

Chapter 33

Bilous, R.W., Donnelly, R., and Idris, I. (2021). *Handbook of Diabetes*, 5e. London: Wiley.

Boore, J., Cook, N., and Shepherd A., (2018). *Essentials of Anatomy and Physiology for Nursing Practice*. London: Sage.

Gordon, C. (2019). Blood glucose monitoring in diabetes: rationale and procedure. *Br. J. Nurs.* 28 (7): 434–439. doi: 10.12968/bjon.2019.28.7.434. PMID: 30969870.

Joint Formulary Committee (2023). British national formulary 85. BMJ Publishing and the Royal Pharmaceutical Society.

NICE (2022). Type 1 diabetes in adults: diagnosis and management. www.nice.org.uk/guidance/ng17/chapter/Recommendations#diagnosis-and-early-care-plan (accessed 18 May 2022).

Chapter 34

IDF (2021). *IDF Diabetes Atlas 2021*, 10e. International Diabetes Federation https://diabetesatlas.org/atlas/tenth-edition (accessed 18 May 2022).

NICE (2017). Type 2 diabetes: prevention in people at high risk (PH38) www.nice.org.uk/guidance/ph38/chapter/Recommendations#risk-assessment (accessed 30 May 2022).

NICE (2022). Type 2 diabetes in adults: management [NG28]. www.nice.org.uk/guidance/ng28/chapter/Recommendations (accessed 31 May 2022).

Chapter 35

Daly, M. and Robinson, E. (2021) Psychological distress associated with the second COVID-19 wave: prospective evidence from the UK household longitudinal study. PsyArXiv.

Long, D., Long, B., and Koyfman, A. (2017). The emergency medicine management of severe alcohol withdrawal. *Am. J. Emerg. Med.* 35: 1005–1011.

World Health Organization (WHO) (2020). Mental disorders. https://www.who.int/news-room/fact-sheets/detail/mental-disorders (accessed 20 November 2022).

Chapter 36

NICE (2019). Diverticular disease: diagnosis and management. www.nice.org.uk/guidance/ng147/chapter/recommendations#diverticular-disease-3 (accessed 20 November 2022).

Peate, I. (2016). *Medical-Surgical Nursing at a Glance (Nursing and Healthcare)*. London: Wiley.

Reichert, M.C. and Lammert, F. (2015). The genetic epidemiology of diverticulosis and diverticular disease: emerging evidence. *United European Gastroenterol. J* 3 (5): 409–418.

Yoon, P., Rajasekar, G., Nuño, M. et al. (2022). Severe obesity contributes to worse outcomes after elective colectomy for chronic diverticular disease. *J. Gastrointest. Surg.* 26 (7): 1472–1481.

Chapter 37

National Institute for Health and Care Excellence (2021). Epilepsies: diagnosis and management. www.nice.org.uk/guidance/cg137 (accessed 22 April 2022).

Scottish Intercollegiate Guidelines Network (2018). Diagnosis and management of epilepsy in adults. A National Clinical Guideline. www.sign.ac.uk/media/1079/sign143_2018.pdf (accessed 22 April 2022).

World Health Organization (2022). Epilepsy. http://www.who.int/news-room/fact-sheets/detail/epilepsy (accessed 22 April 2022).

Chapter 38

NICE (2018). Chronic heart failure in adults: diagnosis and management guideline [NG106]. www.nice.org.uk/guidance/ng106 (accessed 20 November 2022).

Chapter 39

British National Formulary/NICE (2022). HIV infection. HIV infection | Treatment summary | BNF content published by NICE (accessed 22 March 2022).

British Medical Journal (2022). HIV infection. https://bestpractice.bmj.com/topics/en-gb/555 (accessed 22 March 2022).

Daly, M. and Robinson, E. (2021). Psychological distress associated with the second COVID-19 wave: prospective evidence from the UK Household Longitudinal Study. PsyArXiv.

National Institute for Health and Care Excellence (NICE) (2022). Cabotegravir and rilpivirine for treating HIV-1 [ID3766]. Lead team presentation. www.nice.org.uk/guidance/ta757/documents/1 (accessed 22 March 2022).

Steptoe, A. and Di Gessa, G. (2021). Mental health and social interactions of older people with physical disabilities in England during the COVID-19 pandemic: a longitudinal cohort study. *Lancet Public Health* 6 (6): e365–e373.

Tseng, A., Seet, J., and Phillips, E. (2015). The evolution of three decades of antiretroviral therapy: challenges, triumphs and the promise of the future. *Br. J. Clin. Pharmacol.* 79 (2): 182–194.

World Health Organization (WHO) (2020). Mental disorders. https://www.who.int/news-room/fact-sheets/detail/mental-disorders (accessed 20 November 2022).

Chapter 40

BHF (2022). High blood pressure – symptoms and treatment. https://www.bhf.org.uk/informationsupport/risk-factors/high-blood-pressure/symptoms-and-treatment (accessed 20 November 2022).

NHS (2022). Hypertension. https://www.nhs.uk/conditions/high-blood-pressure-hypertension/ (accessed 20 November 2022).

Peate, I. (2022). *Fundamentals of Pathophysiology*, 4e. Oxford: Wiley.

WHO (2021). Hypertension. https://www.who.int/news-room/fact-sheets/detail/hypertension (accessed 20 November 2022).

Chapter 41

Crohn's and Colitis Foundation (2019). Inflammatory bowel disease vs. irritable bowel syndrome. https://www.crohnscolitisfoundation.org/sites/default/files/2019-10/ibd-and-IBS-brochure-final.pdf (accessed 21 November 2022).

Crohn's and Colitis UK (2021). https://crohnsandcolitis.org.uk/media/pcsn5zoo/crohns-ed-8-with-links.pdf (accessed 21 November 2022).

McErlean, L. (2019). Gastrointestinal disorder. In: *Learning to Care: The Nurse Associate* (ed. I. Peate), 398–414. Edinburgh: Elsevier.

Chapter 42

Huang, W.J., Chen, W.W., and Zhang, X. (2017). Multiple sclerosis: pathology, diagnosis and treatments. *Exp. Ther. Med.* 13 (6): 3163–3166. https://doi.org/10.3892/etm.2017.4410.

NHS (2022). MS. https://www.nhs.uk/conditions/multiple-sclerosis/#:~:text=Multiple%20sclerosis%20(MS)%20is%20a,it%20can%20occasionally%20be%20mild (accessed 20 November 2022).

NICE (2014/2019). Clinical guideline CG186. Multiple sclerosis in adults: management. www.nice.org.uk/guidance/cg186 (accessed 20 November 2022).

MS Society (2022). MS in the UK. www.mssociety.org.uk/what-we-do/our-work/our-evidence/ms-in-the-uk#:~:text=Incidence%20and%20prevalence,people%20are%20diagnosed%20with%20MS (accessed 20 November 2022).

Chapter 43

Dorsey, R., Sherer, T., Okun, M.S., and Bloem, B.R. (2020). *Ending Parkinson's Disease: A Prescription for Action*. London: Hachette.

National Institute for Health and Care Excellence (NICE) (2017). Parkinson's disease in adults: diagnosis and management (NG71). www.nice.org.uk/guidance/ng71 (accessed 28 April 2022).

Parkinson's UK (2018). The incidence and prevalence of Parkinson's in the UK. www.parkinsons.org.uk/professionals/resources/incidence-and-prevalence-parkinsons-uk-report (accessed 20 November 2022).

Chapter 44

Blanchflower, J. and Peate, I. (2021). *Fundamentals of Applied Pathophysiology: An Essential Guide for Nursing and Healthcare Students*, 4e. Oxford: Wiley.

GOV.UK (2022). Social prescribing: applying all our health. https://www.gov.uk/government/publications/social-prescribing-applying-all-our-health/social-prescribing-applying-all-our-health (accessed 20 November 2022).

Kings Fund (2020). What is social prescribing. www.kingsfund.org.uk/publications/social-prescribing (accessed 20 November 2022).

Moffatt et al. (2007). *Leg Ulcer Management*, 1st ed. Wiley-Blackwell.

National institute for Health and Care Excellence (2021). How should I interpret ankle brachial pressure index (ABPI) results? http://cks.nice.org.uk (accessed 6 November 2022).

Wounds, U.K. (2019). *Best Practice Statement: Ankle Brachial Pressure Index (ABPI) in Practice*. London: Omniamed Communications Limited.

Chapter 45

National Institute for Health and Care Excellence (2021). Psoriasis assessment and management of psoriasis. www.nice.org.uk/guidance/cg153/evidence/full-guideline-pdf-188351533 (accessed 22 April 2022).

Psoriasis Association (n.d.) Research results. http://www.psoriasis-association.org.uk/research-results (accessed 22 April 2022).

Stephens, M. (2021). The skin and associated disorders. In: *Fundamentals of Applied Pathophysiology. An Essential Guide for Nursing and Health Care Students*, Ch. 20, (ed. I. Peate), 593–622. Oxford: Wiley.

Chapter 46

NICE (2020). Rheumatoid arthritis in adults: management. NICE guideline [NG100].

NHS (2022). Rheumatoid arthritis. https://www.nhs.uk/conditions/rheumatoid-arthritis (accessed 20 November 2022).

National Rheumatoid Arthritis Society (NRAS) (2023). Rheumatoid Arthritis Supporting Information. https://nras.org.uk/information-support/information (accessed 20 November 2022).

Chapter 47

British Society of Haematology (2021). Management of sickle cell disease in pregnancy. A British Society for Haematology guideline. *Br. J. Haematol.* 194: 980–995.

PHE: Public Health England (2018a) National health service (UK). NHS sickle cell and thalassaemia (SCT) screening programme 2016–2017. https://assets.publishing.service.gov.uk/government/uploads/system/uploads/attachment_data/file/713120/SCT_data_report_2016_to_2017.pdf (accessed 20 November 2022).

PHE: Public Health England (2018b) Sickle cell and thalassaemia screening overview. Sickle cell and thalassaemia screening overview – GOV.UK (www.gov.uk) (accessed 20 November 2022).

Sickle Cell society (2021). About sickle cell. https://www.sicklecellsociety.org/about-sickle-cell (accessed 20 November 2022).

Chapter 48

Coelewij, L. and Curtis, D. (2018). Mini-review: update on the genetics of schizophrenia. *Ann. Hum. Genet.* 82 (5): 239–243.

National Institute for Health and Care Excellence (NICE) (2014). Psychosis and schizophrenia: treatment and management. Clinical guideline 178. http://guidance.nice.org.uk/CG178/ (accessed 20 November 2022).

Rethink (2022). Guide to Schizophrenia. https://www.rethink.org/advice-and-information/about-mental-illness/learn-more-about-conditions/schizophrenia (accessed 20 November 2022).

World Health Organization (2019). ICD-11: international classification of diseases. 11th revision. https://icd.who.int (accessed 20 November 2022).

Chapter 49

Alzheimer's Society (2020). Alzheimer's society's view on demography. www.alzheimers.org.uk/about-us/policy-and-influencing/what-we-think/demography (accessed 22 April 2022).

National Institute for Health and Care Excellence (NICE) (n.d.) Prevent or delay the onset of dementia. www.nice.org.uk/about/what-we-do/into-practice/measuring-the-use-of-nice-guidance/impact-of-our-guidance/niceimpact-dementia/ch1-prevent-or-delay-onset-of-dementia (accessed 22 April 2022).

World Health Organization (2021). Dementia. http://www.who.int/news-room/fact-sheets/detail/dementia (accessed 22 April 2022).

Chapter 50

British Association of Sexual Health and HIV (2017). 2017 interim update of the 2015 BASHH National Guidelines for the Management of the Viral Hepatitides. http://www.bashhguidelines.org/media/1161/viral-hepatitides-2017-update-18-12-17.pdf (accessed 22 April 2022).

British Liver Trust (2022). Hepatitis B. www.britishlivertrust.org.uk/information-and-support/living-with-a-liver-condition/liver-conditions/hepatitis-b (accessed 22 April 2022).

Public Health England (2022). Green Book on immunisation Chapter 18 Hepatitis B. UK Government. http://www.gov.uk/government/publications/hepatitis-b-the-green-book-chapter-18 (accessed 22 April 2022).

Chapter 51

Bainter, P.S. (2019). Visual field test, MedicineNet. MedicineNet. https://www.medicinenet.com/visual_field_test/article.htm (accessed 21 November 2022).

NICE (2022). Glaucoma: diagnosis and management. www.nice.org.uk/guidance/ng81/resources/glaucoma-diagnosis-and-management-pdf-1837689655237 (accessed 21 November 2022).

RNIB (2014a). Eye conditions. www.rnib.org.uk/eye-health/eye-conditions (accessed 21 November 2022).

RNIB (2014b). Key information and statistics on sight loss in the UK. www.rnib.org.uk/professionals/knowledge-and-research-hub/key-information-and-statistics (accessed 21 November 2022).

Chapter 52

NHS England (2018a) Making it happen: case finding and risk stratification. https://www.england.nhs.uk/publication/making-it-happen-case-finding (accessed 21 November 2022).

NHS England (2018b) Making it happen: personalised care and support planning. https://www.england.nhs.uk/publication/making-it-happen-personalised-care-and-support-planning (accessed 21 November 2022).

NHS England (2018c) Making it happen: multi-disciplinary team (MDT) working. https://www.england.nhs.uk/publication/making-it-happen-multi-disciplinary-team-mdt-working (accessed 21 November 2022).

Chapter 53

International Council of Nurses (2012). Closing the gap from evidence to practice. https://tinyurl.com/p3pwfsns (accessed 23 July 2022).

Lynch, C. (2022). *Research in Action: The Impact of A Research Placement on Student Nurses' Use of Evidence in Clinical practice*. University of West London.

Rafferty, A.M. (1996). *The Politics of Nursing Knowledge*. London: Taylor & Francis.

Chapter 54

NHS England (2020). Our NHS people. https://www.england.nhs.uk/ournhspeople (accessed 20 November 2022).

NHS Leadership Academy (2014). Healthcare leadership model. https://www.leadershipacademy.nhs.uk/wp-content/uploads/2014/10/NHSLeadership-LeadershipModel-colour.pdf (accessed 20 November 2022).

RCN (2022). Leadership. www.rcn.org.uk/clinical-topics/Clinical-governance/Leadership (accessed 20 November 2022).

Chapter 55

Ford, C. and Robertson, M. (2021). Analgesics. In: *Fundamentals of Pharmacology for Nursing and Healthcare Students* (ed. B. Hill and I. Peate). West Sussex: Wiley.

NICE (2021). Chronic pain. https://cks.nice.org.uk/topics/chronic-pain (accessed 20 November 2022).

Wheeldon, A. (2019). Pain management. In: *Learning to Care, the Nurse Associate* (ed. I. Peate), 334–346. Edinburgh: Elsevier.

Chapter 56

Gold Standards Framework (2006). Prognostic Indicator Guidance to aid identification of adult patients with advanced disease in the last months/year of life, who are in need of supportive and palliative care. Version 1.24. Prognostic Indicator Paper vs. 1.21. www.goldstandardsframework.org.uk Assessed: 19 May 2022.

National Institute for Health and Care Excellence (NICE) (2016). Multimorbidity: clinical assessment and management. NICE guideline NG46. www.nice.org.uk/guidance/ng56 Assessed: 6 August 2022.

National Institute for Health and Care Excellence (NICE) (2019). End of life care for adults: service delivery. NICE guideline NG142. www.nice.org.uk/guidance/ng142/chapter/Recommendations Assessed: 6 September 2022.

Chapter 57

Mental Capacity Act (2005). *Code of Practice (2007)*. London: TSO.

Montaigne, D.M. (1993). *The Complete Essays* (transl. M.A. Screech). London: Penguin Books.

NHS England (2018). My future wishes: advance care planning for people with dementia in all care settings. https://www.england.nhs.uk/publication/my-future-wishes-advance-care-planning-acp-for-people-with-dementia-in-all-care-settings (accessed 23 May 2022).

National Institute for Health and Care Excellence (NICE) (2019). Advanced care planning. A quick guide for registered managers of care homes and home care services. https://www.nice.org.uk/about/nice-communities/social-care/quick-guides/advance-care-planning (accessed 27 March 2023).

Index

Note: Page numbers followed by "*f*" and "*t*" indicate figures and tables, respectively.

abdominal pain and IBD, 97
accountability for health, 29
acquired immune deficiency syndrome (AIDS), HIV and, 92*t*, 93
action stage of behavioural change, 15
active patient participation, 33
activities of daily living (ADL), 133
acute arterial thrombus, 103
acute chest syndrome, 109
acute hepatitis, 115
adapted housing, 11
addiction, 82*f*
    alcohol, 39
    in bipolar disorder and substance misuse, 53
advanced care planning (ACP), 132*t*, 133. *See also* care delivery
        frameworks; end-of-life care (EoLC)
Advanced Decision to Refuse Treatment (ADRT), 133
age-related macular degeneration (AMD), 116*t*, 117
age of individual, 3
agoraphobia, 48*f*, 49
air pollutants, 7
alanine aminotransferase (ALT), 71
alcohol dependency, 38*f*, 39
Alcohol harm identification test (AUDIT), 39
Alcohol IBA screening method, 39
alcoholism, 39
Alcohol use disorder (AUD), 39
Allergy Injectables, 45
α1-antitrypsin, 67
alveolar hypoventilation, 67
Alzheimer's disease, 112*t*, 113, 130
amyloid, 91
amyloidosis, 91
anaemia, 97, 107
anal canal, 84*t*
angina pain, 46*f*, 47
angina pectoris. *See* angina pain
angioplasty with stent. *See* percutaneous coronary intervention
        (PCI)
anhedonia, 111
ankle brachial pressure index (ABPI), 103
ankylosing spondylitis, 42*t*
anorexia-nervosa-focused family therapy (FT-AN), 41
anorexia nervosa, 40*t*, 41, 54
anticholinergics, 130*t*
anticoagulants for atrial fibrillation, 51
anti-convulsant drugs, 53
anti-emetics, 130*t*
anti-psychotic medication for schizophrenia, 111

anti-psychotics, 53
antiretroviral therapy (ART), 93
anxiety, 48*f*, 49
arteries, 102–103
arteriogram, 103
arterioles, 103
arthritis, 42*t*, 43
ascending colon, 84*t*
aspartate aminotransferase (AST), 71
aspirin for diverticular disease, 86
asthma, 6*t*, 45
    pathophysiology of, 44*f*, 45
    patients at risk of developing near-fatal or fatal, 44*t*
    self-management, 29
atherosclerosis, 47
    and CAD, 68*f*, 69
    and PAD, 103
atrial extrasystoles, 51
atrial fibrillation (AF), 50*f*, 50*t*, 50–51
atrial flutter, 51
attachment inhibitors, 92*t*
authoritarian leadership. *See* autocratic leadership
autocratic leadership, 125

behavioural change, 15, 22–23
behavioural risk factors, 8
bereavement, 131
binge eating disorder, 54
bipolar affective disorder, 52–53
bi-polar disorder, 72*f*
bleeding and IBD, 97
blood flow, 62*f*, 63
blood pressure (BP), 95
bradykinesia, 100*t*
bronchiectasis, 56–57
bronchitis, 66*f*, 67
B-type natriuretic peptide (BNP), 91
bulimia-nervosa-focused family therapy (FT-BN), 55
bulimia nervosa, 41, 54–55
bureaucratic leadership, 125
burnout of caregiver, 31

caecum, 84*t*
calcium pyrophosphate disease, 42*t*
calf muscle and foot pumps, 62*t*, 63
calorie intake, 41
cancer, 6*t*, 58–59
capillaries, 102

Long-term Conditions in Adults at a Glance, First Edition. Edited by Aby Mitchell, Barry Hill, and Ian Peate.
© 2023 John Wiley & Sons Ltd. Published 2023 by John Wiley & Sons Ltd.

cardiac:
    amyloidosis, 91
    catheterisation, 91
    MRI, 91
    or valve conditions, 51
    syndrome X. *See* microvascular angina
cardiopulmonary resuscitation (CPR), 133
cardiorespiratory disease, 57
cardiovascular diseases (CVD), 6*t*, 47, 68*f*
cardioversion for atrial fibrillation, 51
care. *See also* advanced care planning (ACP)
    staff, 121
    triangle of, 30*f*
Care Act (2014), 3, 121
care delivery frameworks. *See also* advanced care planning (ACP);
    end-of-life care (EoLC)
    Leading Change, Adding Value framework, 120*f*, 121
    NHS-funded Nursing Care, 121
    NHS Continuing Healthcare, 121
    person-centred care framework, 121
    social care for older people with multiple LTCs, 120*t*, 121
caregiver burnout, 31
Care Quality Commission (CQC), 35
carers, 31
    emotional impact of caring, 31
    supporting, 30*f*, 31
    well-being model, 30*f*
cataract, 116*t*, 117
catheter ablation for atrial fibrillation, 51
CEAP system, 63, 64
childhood arthritis, 43
childhood respiratory disease, 57
Child–Pugh scoring system, Model for End-Stage Liver Disease
    (MELD), 71
children:
    arthritis in, 43
    psychological treatment for bulimia nervosa, 55
cholesterol, 47
chronic alcohol misuse (CAM), 71
chronic fatigue syndrome (CFS), 60*t*, 60*f*, 61
chronic illness, health education using in, 25
chronic ischaemia, 103
chronic liver disease (CLD), 70*f*, 71
chronic obstructive lung disease (COPD), 6*t*, 29, 67
    causes, 67
    chronic bronchitis, 66*f*, 67
    emphysema, 66*f*, 67
    exacerbation of, 67
    MRC dyspnoea scale, 66*t*
    pathophysiology, 67
    self-management, 29
    symptoms, 66*t*, 67
chronic pain, 127
    assessment domains, 126*f*, 127
    causes of, 127
    management, 127
    non-pharmacological strategies, 127*f*, 128
    pain pathway, 126*f*
    pharmacological strategies, 126*f*, 128
chronic venous insufficiency (CVI), 63–64
cirrhosis, 71
co-morbidity, 83
co-receptor antagonists, 92*t*

coaching skills in health education for patients, 24*f*, 25
cognitive behaviour therapy for CFS, 61
colectomy, 86
collective leadership, 125
common mental health disorders (CMD), 8
congestive heart failure, 91
contemplation of behavioural change, 15
continuous glucose monitoring (CGM), 75–76
continuous syringe pumps, 131
coronary angiogram. *See* cardiac—catheterisation
coronary artery disease (CAD), 46*f*, 68*f*, 69
coronary artery spasm. *See* vasospastic angina
coronary heart disease (CHD), 69
corticosteroids, 45
COVID-19 pandemic, 49
    anxiety and depression disorders during, 89
    and SCD, 109
Critical Appraisal Skills Programme, 123
Crohn's disease, 96*f*, 97
cyclothymia, 72*f*
cylindrical bronchiectasis, 56*t*
cystic bronchiectasis, 56*t*
cystic fibrosis, 57
cytokines, 45, 69, 85

death, 131
delusions, 110
dementia, 112–113. *See also* schizophrenia
    causes of, 113
    clinical features, 113
    diagnosis, 113
    with Lewy bodies, 112*t*, 113
democratic leadership, 125
Department of Health and Social Care (DHSC), 133
depression, 52, 72*f*, 73
depressive disorders, 73
descending colon, 84*t*
DESMOND, 80
determinants of health, 3, 4*t*, 5
diabetes mellitus, 29. *See also* type 1 diabetes mellitus (T1DM); type
    2 diabetes mellitus (T2DM)
diabetes prevention programme (DPP), 80
diabetic ketoacidosis (DKA), 75*b*
diabetic retinopathy, 116*t*, 117
Diagnostic and Statistical Manual III (DSM III), 52
dietary and lifestyle factors, 51
direct-acting anticoagulants for atrial fibrillation, 51
discrimination, 5
disease-modifying anti-rheumatic drugs (DMARDs), 43
disease modifying drugs (DMDs), 99
disease modifying therapies (DMTs), 99
diverticular disease, 84
    complications associated with, 85*t*
    diverticular pouch, 85*f*
    key terminology, 84*t*
    risk factors, 84–85
    signs and symptoms, 85–86
    treatment and management, 86
diverticulitis, 84
do not attempt cardiopulmonary resuscitation decisions
    (DNACPR), 133
Doppler testing, 103
Driver and Vehicle Licencing Agency (DVLA), 88*t*, 89

dual diagnosis, 82*f*, 83
dysthymia, 72*f*

eating disorders, 40*t*, 41, 54
echocardiogram for heart failure, 91
education:
  EbE in, 35
  health, 25
  impacts of determinants on health, 4*t*
ejection fraction (EF) for heart failure, 91
elastic arteries, 103
electrocardiogram (ECG):
  angina diagnosis, 47
  for heart failure, 91
electroconvulsive therapy, 73
embolism, 103
emergency medical need, 10*t*
emotional impact of caring, 31
emphysema, 66*f*, 67
end-of-life care (EoLC), 130. *See also* care delivery frameworks
  actively dying phase, 131
  death, 131
  gold standards framework, 130
  indicators of, 130
  symptoms of, 131
  therapeutic medications in, 130*t*
endocrine disrupting chemicals, 7
energy management for CFS, 61
environment, 4*t*
environmental conditions of individual, 3
environmental exposure, 6, 8
environmental factors, 6
  LTCs, 6*f*, 6–7
  physical factors, 7
  psycho-social factors, 7–8
environmental health, 7
epilepsy, 88*f*, 88*t*, 88*b*, 89
Equality Act (2010), 11, 89, 105
evidence-based practice, 123
  barriers to nurses, 123
  hierarchy of evidence, 122*f*, 123
  knowledge translation, 123
  nurse education, 123
  quality appraisal of evidence, 122*t*
exacerbation of COPD, 67
Experts by Experience (EbE), 35
  in clinical practice, 35
  in education, 35
  person-centred care model, 34*f*
  in research and audit, 35
  role in LTC, 35
extra-articular features, 107
extra-cellular matrix, 69
eye function, 117

faecal urgency and IBD, 97
fibrin cuff theory, 64
fistulas, 97
five-year forward view (FYFV), 120*t*, 121
flare-ups/relapse management for CFS, 61
Focal Psychodynamic Therapy (FPT), 41
focal seizures, 89
frequent diarrhoea and IBD, 97
frontotemporal dementia, 112*t*, 113

fusion inhibitors (FIs), 92*t*

gabapentinoids, 128
generalised anxiety disorder (GAD), 48*f*, 49
generalised seizures, 89
geographical characteristics, 7
glaucoma, 116*t*, 117
Global Initiative for Chronic Obstructive Lung Disease (GOLD), 67
glyceryl trinitrate (GTN), 47
gout, 42*t*
graded exercise therapy (GET), 61
gut narrowing, 97

haemoglobin (Hb), 109
hallucinations, 110
haloperidol, 53
'hands-off' leadership. *See* laissez-faire leadership
haustra, 84*t*
HbA1c (glycated haemoglobin), 75, 80
  patient decision aid, 79*f*
  targets, 78*t*
health:
  deal for, 26*f*, 27
  dimensions of, 25
  and home, 11
  inequalities, 3, 4, 5
  promotion, 25
health-care professionals (HCPs):
  using chronic pain assessments, 127
  role in ACP, 133
  role in anxiety disorders, 49
  role in behavioural change, 23
  role in ME/CFS, 61
health education, 25
  coaching skills to patients, 24*f*, 25
  Kirkpatrick model in diabetic patients, 24*t*, 25
  patient-related or nurse-related barriers, 24*t*
  systemic strategies to improve, 25
Health Education England (HEE), 124
Health Research Authority (HRA), 35
Health Survey for England, 39
heart, 62*t*, 63
  failure, 90*f*, 90*t*, 91
  self-management and heart conditions, 29
hepatitides, 114*t*
hepatitis, 114*t*, 115
  hepatitis A, 114*t*, 115
  hepatitis B, 114*t*, 115
  hepatitis C, 114*t*, 115
  hepatitis D, 114*t*, 115
  hepatitis E, 114*t*, 115
hepatitis B surface antibody (HBsAb), 115
hepatocellular jaundice (HCJ), 71
high blood pressure. *See also* hypertension
highly active antiretroviral therapy (HAART), 93
histamine, 45
HIV (human immunodeficiency virus), 93
  and AIDS, 92*t*
  long-acting therapy, 93
  medicines, 92*t*
  stigma and, 93
  supporting those with, 93
  treatments, 92*f*, 93
holism, 18*f*, 19

holistic needs assessment, 18
   House of Care, 18*f*, 19
   self-care and self-management, 18*f*, 19
home, health and, 11
House of Care, 18*f*, 19
housing, 4*t*, 10*t*, 10*f*, 11
hypercortisolaemia, 73
hypertension (HYP), 6*t*, 95
   and cancer, 59
   symptoms of, 94*t*
hypoglycaemia, 75
hypomania, 52
hypophosphatemia, 41
hypoxia, 57, 64, 67

ibuprofen for diverticular disease, 86
ileocaecal sphincter, 84*t*
impaired awareness of hypoglycaemia (IAH), 75
implantable cardioverter defibrillators (ICDs), 131
income, 4*t*
Individual Eating-Disorder-focused Cognitive Behavioural
   Therapy (CBT ED), 41
inflammatory bowel disease (IBD), 97
   causes of, 97
   Crohn's disease, 96*f*, 97
   diagnostic procedures for, 96*t*
   ulcerative colitis, 96*f*, 97
inflammatory vascular disease, 103
inhaled long-acting bronchodilator, 45
inhaled mast cell stabilisers, 45
insulin, 75
   functioning of, 74*f*
   therapies, 74*t*
integrase strand transfer inhibitors (INSTIs), 92*t*
integrated treatment approach, 82*f*, 83
intermediate group of cancer, 59
intermittent claudication, 103
irritable bowel syndrome (IBS), 97
ischaemic heart disease, 130

jaundice, 71
joint pain and destruction of cartilage, 106*f*

kinins, 45
Kirkpatrick model in diabetic patients, 24*t*, 25
knowledge translation, 123

laissez-faire leadership, 125
large intestine, 84*f*, 84*t*
lasting power of attorney (LPA), 133
leadership, 124
   dimensions of, 124*t*, 125
   organisational culture, 125
   styles, 124, 125
Leading Change, Adding Value framework, 120*f*, 121
Leicester Risk Assessment Score 80
less urgent medical need, 10*t*
leukotriene modifiers, 45
lifestyle factors, 3, 14*t*, 14*f*, 14–15
long-acting beta2-agonists (LABAs), 45
long-acting muscarinic antagonists (LAMAs), 45
longer-term survival group of cancer, 59
long-term conditions (LTCs), 6, 6*f*, 8
   and behavioural risk factors, 22

cancer and, 59
EbE role in, 35
and House of Care, 18*f*, 19
linked to behavioural factors, 13
patient empowerment in, 32–33
prevalence in England, 6, 6*f*
and risk factors, 6*t*
self-care, 29
self-management and, 18*f*, 19, 28*t*, 29
and socioeconomic status, 16*f*, 17
low-density lipoprotein (LDL), 47, 69
lung disease and rheumatoid arthritis, 107

Making Every Contact Count (MECC), 12*f*, 13, 23
mania, 52
Maudsley Anorexia Nervosa Treatment for Adults (MANTRA), 41
mechanical theory, 64
medical assessment and housing, 11
medical priority bands, 10*t*
Medical Research Council (MRC) dyspnoea scale, 66*t*
mental health, 82*f*
metre dose inhalers (MDIs), 45
microvascular angina, 47
midwifery, 121
mixed dementia, 113
monoamine neurotransmitter, 73
mood stabilisers, 53
motivational interviewing techniques (MI techniques), 22*t*, 23
mouth ulcers and IBD, 97
mucus and IBD, 97
multifocal atrial tachycardia, 51
multi-infarct dementia, 113
multi-morbidity, 17, 59
multiple sclerosis (MS), 98*t*, 98*f*, 99
muscular arteries, 103
myalgic encephalomyelitis (ME). *See* chronic fatigue syndrome
   (CFS)
My Diabetes My Care, 35
myocardial biopsy, 91
myocardial infarction (MI), 91

National Health Service (NHS), 23
   Constitution for England, 27
   Continuing Healthcare, 121
   high blood pressure, 95
   key principles, 26*b*
   Leadership Academy, 125
   NHS-funded Nursing Care, 121
   patient empowerment, 33
   People Plan, 125
   Plan/Long Term Plan, 3
   providers, 19
   and supporting carers, 31
   Wanless report, 23
National Institute for Health and Care Excellence (NICE), 53, 101,
   111, 121, 133
National Rheumatoid Arthritis Society (NRAS), 107
National Society for Marketing Behaviour, 25
National Statistics Socioeconomic Classification, 16*t*, 17
neurodegenerative disorder, 6*t*
neurotransmitter, 73
noise pollution, 7
non-cardiac conditions, 51
non-diabetic hyperglycaemia (NDH), 80

non-nucleoside reverse transcriptase inhibitors (NNRTIs), 92*t*

noradrenaline, 73

N-terminal pro-brain natriuretic peptide (NT-proBNP), 91

nucleoside reverse transcriptase inhibitors (NRTIs), 92*t*, 93

nurses/nursing, 25, 121

    education, 123

    nurse-related barriers in health education, 24*t*

obesity, 71. *See also* type 1 diabetes mellitus (T1DM); type 2 diabetes mellitus (T2DM)

obsessive compulsive disorder (OCD), 48*f*, 49

occupational and socioeconomic risk factors, 8

olanzapine, 53

oral corticosteroids, 45

organisational culture, 125

osteoarthritis, 43, 43

osteoporosis, 45

other specified feeding or eating disorders (OFSED), 41, 54

pacemakers, 51, 131

pain, 127, 130*t*. *See also* chronic pain

    abdominal, 97

    angina, 46*f*, 47

    and SCD, 109

palliative care, 130

panic attack, 48*f*

panic disorder, 48*f*, 49

Parkinsonism, 101

Parkinson's disease, 100*t*, 101

participative leadership. *See* democratic leadership

particulate matter (PM 2. 5), 7

patient-related barriers in health education, 24*t*

patient empowerment in long-term conditions, 32*f*, 33

patient knowledge, education, and health literacy, 33

patient responsibility, 26–27, 26*f*, 26*b*

percutaneous coronary intervention (PCI), 47

perforation, 97

perinatal depression, 72*f*

peripheral arterial disease (PAD), 102*f*, 102*t*, 103

persistent depressive disorder. *See* dysthymia

person-centred care framework, 121

personal control of patient, 33

personalised patient participation, 33

portal hypertension (PH), 71

post-traumatic stress disorder (PTSD), 48*f*

pre-contemplation of behavioural change, 15

pre-diabetes. *See* non-diabetic hyperglycaemia (NDH)

prevent, protect, and promote of public health (3 Ps), 12*f*, 13

Primary Care Mortality Database (PCMD), 69

primary progressive MS, 98*t*

Prinzmetal's angina. *See* vasospastic angina

prodromal non-motor features of Parkinson's disease, 101

prodromal phase of schizophrenia, 110

prostaglandins, 45

protease inhibitors (PIs), 92*t*, 93

prothrombin time (PT), 71

pruritis, 105

psoriasis, 104*f*, 104*b*, 105

psoriatic arthritis, 42*t*, 105

psycho-education, 111

psycho-social interventions, 111

psychotic depression, 72*f*

public health, 12*f*, 13

pulmonary vasoconstriction, 67

quetiapine, 53

Rainbow model, 3

reactive arthritis, 42*t*

reactive depression, 72*f*

Recommended Summary Plan for Emergency Care and Treatment document (ReSPECT document), 133

recurrent depression, 72*f*

red blood cell (RBC), 109

relapses, 15

    prevention programme, 83

    remitting MS, 98*t*

research and audit, EbE in, 35

Resist, Understand, Listening and Empower (RULE), 23

respirator pump, 62*t*

respiratory acidosis, 67

respiratory muscle fatigue, 67

retina, 117

rheumatoid arthritis (RA), 106*t*, 107

rheumatoid arthritis, 43

rigidity, 100*t*

risperidone, 53

saccular bronchiectasis, 56*t*

schizophrenia, 110–111

seasonal affective disorder, 72*f*

sedatives, 130*t*

seizure, 88*f*, 89

selective mutism, 48*f*, 49

self-care, 19, 29, 33

self-efficacy of patient, 33

self-management, 28*t*, 29

    and long-term conditions, 18*f*, 19

    skills, 33

    stages and indicators of empowerment, 32*f*

septic arthritis, 43

serotonin, 73

shared responsibilities of patients, 26*b*, 27

short-acting anticholinergics, 45

short-acting beta2-agonists (SABAs), 45

shorter-term survival group, 59

sickle cell, 108*f*

sickle cell anaemia, 109

sickle cell crisis, 109

sickle cell disease (SCD), 108*t*, 109

sickle C thalassaemia, 109

sickle thalassaemia. *See* sickle C thalassaemia

sight loss. *See* visual impairment

sigmoid colon, 84*t*

single-infarct dementia, 113

sinus rhythm, 51

sinus tachycardia, 51

situational leadership, 125

six steps approach to ACP, 132*t*

skin, 105

    changes in PAD, 103

    disease, 105

sleep disturbance, 7

smooth muscle cells (SMC), 69

Snellen chart, 117

social anxiety, 48*f*

social capital interventions, 8

social care for older people with multiple LTCs, 120*t*, 121

social class, 16*t*, 17

social determinants of health, 5
social environment, 7–8
social justice, 4f, 5, 8
social marketing in health education, 25
social prescribing, 29
socioeconomic classification, 17
socioeconomic position. *See* socioeconomic status
socioeconomic status, 16t, 16f, 17
Specialist Supportive Clinical Management (SSCM), 41
specific phobias, 48f
stable angina, 47
steatosis, 71
stepped care approach, 49
steroids, 43
stiff heart syndrome. *See* cardiac amyloidosis
stigma and HIV, 93
stroke:
    and self-management, 29
    stroke-related dementia, 113
subcortical dementia, 113
subcutaneous immunotherapy (SCIT), 45
substance abuse, 83
supraventricular tachycardias, 51

T1D. *See* type 1 diabetes mellitus (T1DM)
T2D. *See* type 2 diabetes mellitus (T2DM)
temporary lapse stage, 15
tobacco smoke, 67
toxic mega colon, 97
transactional leadership, 125
transformational leadership, 125
transport, 4t
transtheoretical model of behavioural change, 15
transverse colon, 84t
'trap' growth factor theory, 64
tremor, 100t
triglycerides, 47
type 1 bipolar disorder, 53
type 1 diabetes mellitus (T1DM), 74f, 74–76

type 2 bipolar disorder, 53
type 2 diabetes (T2DM), 71
type 2 diabetes mellitus (T2DM), 6t, 71, 78t, 78f, 79–80

UK National Screening Committee (UK NSC), 109
ulcerative colitis, 96f, 97
United Kingdom Model for End-Stage Liver Disease (UKELD), 71
unstable angina, 47
urgent medical need, 10t

vascular dementia, 112f, 112t, 113
vascular smooth muscle cell (VSMC) migration, 69
vaso-occlusive crisis, 109
vasospastic angina, 47
veins, 62t, 63
venous system, 62t, 63
ventricular ectopic beats, 51
viral hepatitis, 115
visual acuity (VA), 117
visual impairment:
    eye conditions causing, 116t
    pharmacology, 117
vitamin D deficiency in UK, 7

Wanless report to behavioural change, 23
warfarin for atrial fibrillation, 51
weight loss and IBD, 97
well-being:
    health and, 3
    housing and, 11
    impacts of, 4t
white blood cell theory, 64
World Health Organization (WHO), 6
    and asthma, 45
    AUDIT, 39
    and bipolar affective disorder, 53
    data of LTCs, 6
    dimensions of health, 25
    and hypertension, 95